The influences of religion in the history of the United States are complex and messy. This book is unique in examining those influences in the context of America's global health and development programs and priorities. For those of us working in the fields of public health and development, it reminds us of a history that we've largely forgotten but has lingering consequences; such a reminder equips us to better understand the ongoing influences of religion in our work today and helps us plan and execute our efforts with heightened awareness and sensitivity.

– Sandra Thurman, Chief Strategy Officer in The Office of the U.S. Global AIDS Coordinator and Health Diplomacy, USA

This book explores how Christianity has influenced America's role in global health and development over the course of our nation's existence. The ubiquitous but ever-changing influence of religion illuminates how it combines with scientific and social aspects to provide social good, but also cause potential harm. It is a must read for those concerned with global health policy.

– James Curran, Dean, Rollins School of Public Health, Emory University, USA

John Blevins has given us a history of the role of American Protestantism as a formative influence on the structures of faith-based organizations that work in the world of global public health and community development. American Protestantism's deep flaws and soaring accomplishments are on full display in this history of its outreach to many cultures and its building of schools and hospitals around the world. Blevins' highly original account brings together both familiar and unfamiliar individuals and helpfully offers us a framework for seeing their work, and the institutions that have resulted from it as evangelism, engineering, and reconstruction. Blevins, who is both a scholar and a practitioner, concludes with a fair-minded assessment of what we should know, and do—now—to promote global health.

– Ellen Idler, Samuel Candler Dobbs Professor of Sociology, and Director, Religion and Public Health Collaborative, Emory University, USA

This masterful work is a pathbreaking contribution to the growing scholarship on the role of religion in global health and development practices. This social history fills a major gap in our understanding by skillfully tracing the history of American Protestantism's involvement in this complex and contested set of issues. Anyone interested in the multivalent role of religion in global affairs has to read this book.

– Shaun Casey, Director of the Berkley Center for Religion, Peace, and World Affairs, Georgetown University, USA

Christianity's Role in United States Global Health and Development Policy

In recent years, researchers and practitioners in global health and development have shown a renewed interest in religion. In many instances, their interest has focused on ways to ensure that the contributions and capacities of faith-based organizations are maximized in achieving global health and development objectives. There are, however, other critical questions to be asked in regard to religion's influence on global health and development. This book offers a sustained social and political history that helps to illuminate some of those questions. *Christianity's Role in United States Global Health and Development Policy: To Transfer the Empire of the World* examines the role of American Protestantism in making possible the first examples of global health initiatives carried out through medical missions and in influencing the idea that America has both the responsibility and the authority to intervene in other parts of the world for the good of the people there.

Beginning in the colonial era of the nation and continuing up to the present, this book surveys 300 years of social, political, and religious movements through the lens of global health and development. This book is not an apologetics for this distinctly American form of Christianity but a critical history of Christianity in America that demonstrates both the benefits and costs of religion in these fields. Researchers from across global health, politics, history, religion, and development studies will be interested in the wide-ranging questions posed by this book.

John Blevins is an Associate Research Professor and Acting Director of the Interfaith Health Program at the Hubert Department of Global Health, Rollins School of Public Health, Emory University, USA.

Routledge Research in Religion and Development

The *Routledge Research in Religion and Development* series focuses on the diverse ways in which religious values, teachings, and practices interact with international development.

While religious traditions and faith-based movements have long served as forces for social innovation, it has only been within the last ten years that researchers have begun to seriously explore the religious dimensions of international development. However, recognizing and analyzing the role of religion in the development domain are vital for a nuanced understanding of this field. This interdisciplinary series examines the intersection between these two areas, focusing on a range of contexts and religious traditions.

Religion and Urbanism
Reconceptualising sustainable cities for South Asia
Yamini Narayanan

Religions and Development in Asia
Sacred Places as Development Spaces
Matthew Clarke and Anna Halahoff

Between Humanitarianism and Evangelism in Faith-based Organisations
A Case from the African Migration Route
May Ngo

Christianity's Role in United States Global Health and Development Policy
To Transfer the Empire of the World
John Blevins

Christianity's Role in United States Global Health and Development Policy

To Transfer the Empire of the World

John Blevins

Routledge
Taylor & Francis Group
LONDON AND NEW YORK

First published 2019
by Routledge
2 Park Square, Milton Park, Abingdon, Oxon OX14 4RN

and by Routledge
711 Third Avenue, New York, NY 10017

Routledge is an imprint of the Taylor & Francis Group, an informa business

British Library Cataloguing-in-Publication Data
A catalog record for this book is available from the British Library

Library of Congress Cataloging-in-Publication Data
A catalog record for this book has been requested

ISBN: 978-0-8153-5673-8 (hbk)
ISBN: 978-1-351-12750-9 (ebk)

Typeset in Perpetua
by Apex CoVantage, LLC

To our sons, John Brogan and Sam. And to the engineer (Rande), evangelist (Lesley), and reconstructionist (Linda) for your roles in molding them into the young men they are today.

Contents

Tables

Acknowledgments

There is no better place in the world to study the intersection of religion and public health than Emory University. The university has a strong school of public health (including the largest student enrollment in global health in the world), a rigorous religious studies program at both the undergraduate and graduate levels, and a vibrant school of theology that prepares students for vocational ministry in the Christian tradition. Emory is one of the few American research universities that values the contributions of religious study to the intellectual life of the community and takes the study of religion seriously, without dogmatic demands. I am fortunate to have worked with colleagues at Emory in exploring this intersection of religion and public health for over a decade. Emory's Religion and Public Health Collaborative brings together scholars from public health, nursing, medicine, law, religious studies, theology, anthropology, and sociology to carry out interdisciplinary research in the field. Ellen Idler, a sociologist and epidemiologist who has generated a tremendous body of research examining religion's influence on health across the lifespan, is the director of the collaborative; in that role, she has created an environment in which scholars and students from across disciplines can learn from one another and generate a body of scholarship unparalleled anywhere. Since 2009, I have had the good fortune to be part of the Interfaith Health Program (IHP) in the Rollins School of Public Health at Emory. This applied research and practice initiative has been an incubator for innovative initiatives to build on the contributions of religion in support of improved health both in the United States and in various global contexts. Colleagues in IHP have included Sandra Thurman, Susan Landskroener, Aneesah Akbar-Uqdah, Ahoua Kone, and Emily Lemon, in addition to a host of graduate students who have been part of various fieldwork project over the years; I've been enriched by and learned from knowing all of them.

I was introduced to the field of religion and global health and development in 2004 when I volunteered with Lonnie and Fran Turner, two missionaries who have been working alongside women and men in Zambia since the 1970s. In partnership with local communities, the Turners are implementing sustainable agricultural and educational initiatives that have a direct, immediate impact on people's health and well-being. They first helped me to understand the characteristics of such work and the commitments that make it possible.

The field of religion and global health and development is growing rapidly and colleagues both in universities and organizations enrich me with their insights and commitments on an ongoing basis. These colleagues include Jill Olivier, Esther Mombo, Jean Duff, Sally Smith, Julienne Munyaneza, Nyambura Njoroge, and Francesca Merico; I am better in every way for knowing them.

Finally, I want to thank Mimi Kiser at Emory's Interfaith Health Program. For over two decades, Mimi has lived out and held on to the best intentions and commitments in this field. My office is next door to Mimi's, which gives me a front row seat to her energy and passion. It's a wonderful sight in a world that is too often dulled by cynicism and suspicion.

Introduction

In 1800, the Reverend Nathaniel Emmons preached a Thanksgiving Day sermon describing the ways in which God had ordained America as "a peculiar people" to serve as a light unto the other nations of the world, testifying to God's mercy and grace in order that God might bring about a global society bound together in Christian harmony. Emmons's sermon reveals a number of theological, cultural, and political assumptions common to his day: a zeal to convert "the heathens" to Christianity that their souls might be saved from eternal damnation, a sincere belief that missionary efforts also provided an opportunity—no, a responsibility—to export American civilization to other nations in order to fulfill America's providential role as the instrument for ordering human societies and human governments to reflect God's intention and an arrogance to employ the mechanisms of empire to bring about both religious conversion and cultural assimilation:

> We shall soon rise superior to every other kingdom on earth . . . If our present enterprising spirit continues to operate, and the smiles of Heaven continue to attend our vigorous exertions, we shall in a very short time have the possession and dominion of this whole western world. It seems to be the design of Providence to diminish other nations, and to increase and strengthen ours . . . Hence there is great reason to believe that God is about to transfer the empire of the world from Europe to America, where he has planted his peculiar people. And should this be the design of Heaven, we shall undoubtedly continue to spread and increase until we become the most numerous and powerful nation on earth.[1]

Emmons's sermon on that Thanksgiving Day did not merely recite America's civil religion—though it indeed did do that; it also represented his ideas regarding foreign missions. As much as any religious leader of the late eighteenth and early nineteenth centuries in America, Emmons provided a foundation for the nation's emerging missionary zeal. He helped found the Massachusetts Missionary Society in 1800 and served as its president for 12 years. In 1810, he was a founding officer of the American Board of Commissioners for Foreign Missions, a national body of Protestant denominations joining together to support foreign missions initiatives around the world.[2] The religious, cultural, and political world that Emmons envisioned served as one foundation for American practices of global health and development, not only during the decades of Emmons's, life but even up into the present. This book tells the story of that world and offers a 300-year social history on the ways in which religious and secular efforts to care for those in need—first through foreign missions, and later through the health and development programs made possible in American foreign policy—reflected the effort to "transfer the empire of the world."

According to America's religious and political leaders, this transfer has been twofold. First, America became the receptacle of God's providential favor in the face of European societies who had turned away from true faith to ruinous error. In this way, then, these leaders believed that the first transfer had occurred when America chose to be an exemplar—a city on a hill—that reflected God's intention for how society should be structured. Europe had offered a hope for such a structure but had failed to bring it to fruition; America would complete the task. The second transfer would occur as American Christians spread the gospel not only of salvation through Jesus but of the beneficent largesse of the American people to cultures across the world.

This transfer of empire occurred, in part, through global health and development programs carried out by Americans to alleviate the suffering of people in need. The book is not at all justification of such efforts, but, rather, a recounting of the ways that the tentacles of empire can spread not only through the strength of military interventions but through programs that wrap themselves in the practices of religious and secular compassion. Recounting this story is important at this point in time because secular global health and development initiatives have realized the importance of religion in their efforts. After being ignored for over 30 years, religion has once again become a social force that has captured the attention of researchers and practitioners in global health and development. Let's begin by offering some evidence for this renewed interest.

Religion, health, and development by the numbers

In 1640, the Capuchin missionaries of the Roman Catholic Church founded a mission hospital in the nation now known as Angola. The London Missionary Society sent Dr. Johannes Van der Kamp as its first medical missionary to Cape Town in 1795.[3] The foreign missions activities of Christian organizations laid the foundation for modern health care in many parts of the world, with the clearest and longest-landing contributions of those efforts seen in sub-Saharan Africa today. Through the nineteenth and twentieth centuries, Protestant and Catholic missionary bodies established the only health networks of any size across the sub-Saharan region of Africa. In 1890 The Society of the Missionaries of Africa had a network of 46 missionary stations administering a network of 60 hospitals, dispensaries, and orphanages that cared for 344,615 patients. By 1910, they treated 1,219,869 in 289 facilities. Roman Catholic missionaries founded Sacred Heart Hospital, the first hospital in Nigeria in Abeokuta in 1895.[4] Without exception, the only source of dedicated clinical medical practices across the European colonies at the turn of the century came from Christian missionaries.[5]

Today, faith-based health facilities are the largest non-governmental provider of health services across sub-Saharan Africa.[6] They have been essential in addressing the global HIV pandemic; for example, a person living with HIV in either Nairobi or Mombasa—Kenya's two largest cities, both of which have high HIV prevalence—is more likely to get life-saving antiretroviral treatment from a faith-based facility than from any other type, including those managed by the Kenya government.[7]

A new field emerging

Given this history of geographic reach, longevity, and capacity among faith-based facilities, there is little wonder why global health and development practitioners and researchers have had a conversion experience—they have found religion. And they have found religion because they recognize how little they know of its function—a gap in knowledge that is rather problematic given the scope of the services offered by faith-based providers. In fact, the interest in religion is a relatively new phenomenon. Up until a decade ago, many health and development practitioners and researchers minimized the influence of religious beliefs in the lives of the people to whom they provided services, overlooked the importance of partnerships with faith-based health and development programs, and insisted that religious belief remain segregated as a private matter which should have no bearing on health policies.

Today, things have certainly changed. In 2015, at a high-level conference hosted by the World Bank on the importance of faith-based partners to the global development agenda, Jim Yong Kim, President of the World Bank Group, spoke of the importance of his own Roman Catholic faith and the liberation theology tradition within Catholicism as a foundation for his own personal commitment as well as the Bank's institutional commitment to utilize the Bank's resources to address economic disparities:

> The foundation of everything I have done has been through this notion of a preferential option for the poor . . . We looked around the world and asked if there was an approach that made sense, and nothing gave as much clarity as the notion of a preferential option for the poor, and every religion shared that.[8]

Bi-lateral health and development initiatives, such as the U.S. President's Emergency Plan for AIDS Relief (PEPFAR), and multilateral initiatives, such as the Global

Fund to End Malaria, Tuberculosis and HIV (Global Fund), focus on strengthening their faith-based partnerships,[9] and a whole host of United Nations Programs, including the United Nations Development Program (UNDP),[10] the United Nations Joint Programme on HIV/AIDS (UNAIDS),[11] the World Health Organization (WHO),[12] and UNICEF[13] (among others) regularly consult with faith-based partners on furthering the health and development agenda.

Major research universities in the United States now offer courses on religion and public health or religion and development practice, and some of these offer dual-degree graduate programs in public health and theological studies or development practice and theological studies. Yale, Harvard, the University of California at Berkley, Johns Hopkins, Georgetown, Boston, and Emory universities all offer specific coursework in religion and public health or religion and development. Emory, Yale, and Andrews universities offer graduate-level dual degrees in public health and theological studies. Clearly, then, the fields of public health and development practice have found religion.

In fact, this interest in religion is not so much a newly found conversion as a rediscovery. Religious motivations, organizations, beliefs, and practices have had a long, formative impact on present-day frameworks through which global health and development initiatives are carried out. While the religious roots of these frameworks or the influences of religious beliefs and practices on health and development policy may have been played down for the last three decades of the twentieth century, this has been the exception and not the norm over the last three centuries. This book is a social and political history of the intersections of religion and global health and development in the United States during those 300 years. This introduction lays out the focuses and limitations of the work, makes the case for why those focuses are relevant in light of those limitations, discusses the relationship of this book to other research in the field, and provides a brief overview of the book's structure and contents of each chapter.

Focusing on this subject presupposes limitations. The history to be recounted in the pages that follow has a particular religious focus that is Christian—specifically, Protestant Christian—and a cultural and political focus that is American. The reasons for such focuses are straightforward. The cultural and political focus on the United States reflects the sizable influence of American foreign policy on health and development efforts carried out on the global stage, especially over the last century. While other countries influence global health and development initiatives and religion has undoubtedly impacted their global health policies, programs, and priorities, religion nonetheless has impacted U.S global health and development priorities in distinctive ways. Those influences have long historical roots that reach into the present day and impact programs globally because of the social, economic, and political power of the United States, for better or worse. The focus on Protestant Christianity reflects the major, formative role that this tradition has played in shaping America and its religious rhetoric for over three hundred years. In 1927, Andre Siegfried, a leading French political theorist, visited North America in order to understand the social and political forces that were shaping Canada and the United States after the end of the Great War. In his analysis as a French observer of religion's influence on American culture, Siegfried wrote,

> If we wish to understand the real sources of American inspiration, we must go back to the English Puritanism of the seventeenth century, for the civilization of the United States is essentially Protestant. Those who prefer other systems, such as Catholicism, for example, are considered bad Americans and are sure to be frowned on by the purists. Protestantism is the only national religion, and to ignore that fact is to view the country from a false angle.[14]

The America of the twenty-first century undoubtedly has social and religious influences other than Protestantism alone; nonetheless, this book argues American Protestantism was so foundational in establishing the cultural, political, and religious worldview of the United States from the 1600s through the middle 1900s that understanding the nation today requires some knowledge of Protestantism's impact in these earlier generations. There are many texts which analyze Protestantism's influence on various aspects of American society, but there has not been a book-length analysis of its role on setting the global health and development policies championed by the U.S. government.

Although the book focuses on the influence of religion on American foreign policies of health and development, it is not a piece of propaganda or an apologetics of those policies. In fact, the book will examine religion's relationship to the political contexts that shaped the country's international aid and development policies through a critical lens. The focus on Christian Protestantism is necessary because of the influence of this expression of Christianity on the politics of the United States. Such a focus, however, does not presume that Christian Protestantism is the only expression of religion in America, that is "better" or "more true" than other expressions of Christianity (for example, Roman Catholicism), or that it is better or more true than other religious traditions that are part of the nation's religious fabric. In short, this book does not articulate a theological perspective making normative claims about the truth of the Christian religion but a sociological analysis of religion in America in regard to its influence on global health and development; such an analysis in the American context will, of necessity, focus on Christian Protestantism.

This book is part of a rapidly growing body of research and scholarship in religion, health, and development. It both draws from this work and focuses on some critical perspectives that distinguish it from this other work. Scholars and researchers from a variety of disciplines and practitioners working in the fields of health and development have generated an entirely new field of academic inquiry into religion's influence on health and development practice. The majority of this work has advanced the idea that religiously motivated health and development initiatives are essential partners for trusted, sustainable, and effective efforts. Examples of such perspectives can be found in *Sacred Aid*,[15] *Beholden: Religion, Global Health, and Human Rights*,[16] *Religion and the Health of the Public*,[17] and *Spirits of Protestantism*.[18] Other contributions present findings in academic journals in the fields of public health, development practice, and public policy to describe the extent of religion's influence on development and health practice. Examples include a series of articles in *The Lancet*[19] and a special issue in the journal *Development in Practice*.[20] Still others make the case that while religion has often been overlooked, it is, in fact, a powerful social force that needs to be studied—an effort to legitimate the field of religion in global health and development. Examples include the multi-author volume *Religion as a Social Determinant of Public Health*[21] as well as the texts in the Routledge Press series in Research in Religion and Development, a series which includes this volume. A smaller body of research argues that religion complicates and hinders public health and development goals, especially in the context of sexual and reproductive health and HIV/AIDS. Examples include *The Invisible Cure*[22] and policy analyses from research consortiums such as the analysis of U.S. global HIV programs entitled *How Ideology Trumped Science*.[23] Titles in a similar vein carry out a political analysis; these include *Of Little Faith: The Politics of George W. Bush's Faith-Based Initiatives*.[24]

In addition to academic writing, research centers and initiatives have grown in recent years, including the Berkley Center and World Faiths Development Dialogue at Georgetown University; the Religion and Public Health Collaborative and the Interfaith Health Program at Emory University; the International Religious Health Assets Programme at the University of Cape Town; the Joint Learning Initiative on Faith and Local Communities; the Center for Faith and the Common Good; the Religion and International Development Group at the American Academy of Religion; the Religion, Health and Medicine Group at the American Academy of Religion; and the Faith Caucus at the American Public Health Association. While these lists are not intended to be exhaustive, they do demonstrate the recent interest in religion in the fields of public health and development practice.

Distinctive characteristics of this book

This book is part of this emerging body of work, and it differs from it in some noteworthy ways. More often than not, religion has been treated in this body of research in instrumentalist and positivistic ways. An instrumentalist approach to religion focuses on what religion accomplishes or achieves. For those working in the fields of global health and development, a great deal of the new-found interest in religion focuses on what it achieves in regard to health and development programs, services, and capacities. A focus on the instrumentality of religion is seen in research (some of which I have carried out)[25] to determine the percentage of health services provided by faith-based facilities. Such research interests health and development practitioners because it is needed to set priorities, understand the geographic and programmatic reach of partnerships, and build and sustain capacity. A positivistic approach to religion assumes that its relevance to research and applied practice in the field is limited to the aspects of religion that can be measured and assessed. Positivism focuses on the concrete. It conceptualizes "religiosity" through clearly defined metrics; these often include measures such as religious attendance, a content analysis of doctrinal statements or denominational positions, or self-reports of belief in God. Positivism allows for replicability across study sites or a comparative analysis of different studies that each measure religion according to similar metrics such as religious attendance.

Both positivism and instrumentalism are common methods for studying religion in the fields of global health and development but there are problems with both. First of all, these approaches fail to adequately describe religion as a phenomenon. The varied effects of religion—effects which are both simultaneous and contradictory because of their variety—go unexamined. Religious attendance cannot account for negotiations that happen in the lives of people of faith between their attendance at religious services, their own religious beliefs, and their daily life choices beyond religious practice. A content analysis of religious doctrines fails to assess how people inside of a religious tradition may assent to those doctrines as true and valid or reject them even while remaining in the tradition. A second problem, related to the first, is that scholars of religion rarely conceptualize it in instrumentalist or positivistic ways. These conceptual misalignments can complicate interdisciplinary research into religion, health, and development. In one instance, researchers in the health sciences may carry out a multivariate analysis to measure the correlation between religious attendance, self-reports of daily prayer, and clinical markers of hypertension. In another, scholars in religious studies are calling for an a/theological realignment of beliefs following the demise of metaphysics as a defining characteristic of poststructuralism. Trying to find a common thread between these two analyses of this thing we call religion will be frustrating and may possibly be fruitless without collegiality across the disciplines. One can understand just how difficult meaningful interdisciplinary research can be given such disparate fields of reference.

Advocates for religion's potential contributions in the health and development field worked long and hard for over a decade to make the case for religion's contributions in fields that were initially skeptical and non-committal. In doing so, they highlighted religion as an asset to health and development. One wonders, however, if they might have oversold their case. Clearly, religion may be at odds with health and development initiatives; there is ample evidence of this in global HIV programs, for example. Demonstrating that religion is an asset to health and development while minimizing religion's negative effects is not sound scholarship but one-sided apologetics.

This text works hard to avoid either of these approaches. As a social history, it offers numerous instances of religion's influence on health and development without relying on instrumentalist or positivistic frames. In recounting that history, it recounts examples of religion furthering health and development programs and thwarting such initiatives. Further, it assesses the fields of health and development as well, arguing that new critical perspectives are sorely needed. In this way, I hope that this text will be part of a new thread of scholarship and research that can deepen the conceptual richness of religion in the fields of global health and development.

What's in store: the contents of the book

This social history of American Protestantism and its influences on global health and development unfolds across eight chapters. Chapter 1 examines the period from the colonial era to the mid-1800s, when a theological vision of America's providential role in redeeming the world emerged among America's Protestant Christians. The chapter traces the ways in which that vision influenced religious belief and practice, missionary activity, ideas about the purpose of foreign missions, and the politics of the new nation. Chapter 2 examines the ways in which scientific advances and a broader ethos of social reform during the Progressive Era set the stage for new models of foreign missions and public health. It also reveals how the desire to address social ills in these movements was carried out in frameworks that were explicitly racist so that the era is marked both by admirable efforts to reduce social inequities and by an astounding blindness to the assumptions of white, Anglo-Saxon superiority. Politically, America continued its westward expansion and established a more robust—some might even say confrontational—approach to foreign policy based on the idea of American exceptionalism that had its roots in American Christianity.

Chapter 3 examines the first half of the twentieth century. From the turn of the century to the end of the Second World War, American Protestantism exerted tremendous influence on American society, especially through programs of social reform known as the Social Gospel. The Social Gospel movement sought to "Christianize the social order" and key aspects of the movement influenced public health programs and policies, both in the United States and in global contexts. A robust program of foreign missions influenced global health and development practices in the era and also contributed to a number of non-religious initiatives through government and civil society that would set the stage for global health and development efforts in the latter half of the twentieth century.

At the same time, however, disagreements on various social issues led to the fragmentation of a unified vision among a broad cross-section of American Protestants. The reforms of the Social Gospel would not be sustained under that name and liberal Protestantism would wrestle with a crisis of confidence. Nonetheless, many of the Social Gospel ideals would find various institutional homes to influence the United States government's foreign policy priorities. The chapter concludes with a case study of the Rockefeller family as a way to trace these shifts over the decade of the early to mid-twentieth century and to demonstrate the ways in which American Protestantism played a significant role in establishing the field of public health and the federal government's foreign aid programs.

In Chapter 4, the analysis turns to the key elements of Social Gospel principles that migrated beyond Protestant denominations into a variety of global governmental and civil society contexts. This chapter traces that migration using the concepts of social evangelists, social engineers, and social reconstructionists. Social evangelists articulated Social Gospel aims and commitments in the institutions of civil society; this chapter describes the role of religious leaders involved in efforts to establish the United Nations as examples of these evangelists. Social engineers sought to develop, test, and perfect methodologies to carry out global health and development work that would make a measurable difference; this chapter describes Bill Foege's contributions toward the eradication of smallpox and his subsequent efforts at global childhood immunization in partnership with his colleague James Grant at UNICEF as examples of the social engineer. Social reconstructionists focus on a critical analysis of the social and political systems that thwart health and development efforts; the chapter examines the ideas of Ivan Illich regarding clinical, social, and cultural iatrogenesis as an example of social reconstructionism. The fifth chapter continues the analysis begun in Chapter 4 by describing efforts to carry out hybrid models among the three in various combinations. The first hybrid model, the evangelist/engineer, is represented in the work of the Christian Medical Commission (CMC) of the World Council of Churches and the influence of the CMC on the broader primary health care movement championed by the World Health Organization during the 1970s. The second hybrid model, the evangelist/reconstructionist, is represented in the various theologies from Christians both in the United States and around the globe who continued to develop pointed critiques of social and religious forces in order to provide a new framework for Christian theologies of justice. The chapter surveys a number of theological movements and examines the influences of a handful of them in relation to global health and development.

The third hybrid model, the engineer/reconstructionist, is represented by Halfdan Mahler, the Director General of the World Health Organization from 1973–1988. Mahler was unafraid to take seriously the critical ideas of the reconstructionists to overhaul the WHO's priorities through the primary health care movement. The fourth and final hybrid model, the evangelist/engineer/reconstructionist, is represented in the principles set forth in Alma-Ata Declaration on Primary Health Care.

Chapter 6 serves as a reminder that American Protestantism was focused not only on enacting Social Gospel ideals in support of global health and development in the latter part of the twentieth century. The tradition was also used—sometimes willingly and sometimes not—by politicians in the U.S. government to articulate a civil religion during the Cold War. This chapter examines the relationship between mainline Protestants and Presidents Truman and Eisenhower, as well as the first stirrings of a soon-to-be emergent evangelicalism. The chapter also examines the public health response to Cold War threats and the ways in which international aid was used as an instrument to further American interests during the period. The seventh chapter surveys the current religious landscape in America in which mainline Protestantism no longer retains the social influence it once enjoyed. This chapter surveys other Christian traditions—notably, Roman Catholicism and evangelical Protestantism—as well as other religions and the growing influence of the religious "nones," people who identify no denominational or religious affiliation in the United States. The public health and development aspects of each of those traditions are also examined.

In the book's eighth and last chapter, I review the complex ways that religion has intersected with global health and development efforts with mixed results. In recounting various instances touched on earlier in the book, the chapter lays out the argument that the current research interest in religion, health, and development needs to more fully and critically examine religion's varied effects on health and development programs and policies. The chapter also explores the idea that global health and development practice cannot avoid the possibility of tragic outcomes because at times it places practitioners in the field in complex situations in which there is no option to carry out the good without also enabling negative consequences. The chapter argues that in such instances, practitioners in the fields of public health and development studies are ill-equipped to examine the impact of our work because the primary criteria employed for determining whether a project is right are the good effects it produces. Thus, when a project also carries with it negative consequences, those of us working in the fields are unsure what to do. The chapter asks whether one important and distinctive contribution that religion might make in such circumstances would be its ability to provide a history of the limitations of our efforts and the reality of tragic possibilities.

Notes

1 Nathanael Emmons, *A Sermon, Preached on the Annual Thanksgiving in Massachusetts. November 27, 1800* (Wrentham, MA: Nathaniel Heaton, 1801), 19–20.
2 For a description of the importance of missions' efforts to Emmons's ministry, see Jacob Ide, ed. *The Works of Nathaniel Emmons with a Memoir of His Life, Vol. I* (Boston: Congregational Board of Publications, 1861). See especially, chapter 11: "His Connection with the Cause of Missions," pp. 176–200.
3 Charles M. Good, "Pioneer Medical Missions in Africa," in *Social Science and Medicine* 32, no. 1 (1991): 3.
4 Ibid., p. 4.
5 Michael Worboys, "The Colonial World as Mission and Mandate," in *Osiris* 15 (2000): 208.

6 Jill Olivier, Clarence Tsimpo, Regina Gemignani, Mari Shojo, Harold Coulombe, et. al., "Understanding the Roles of Faith-Based Health-Care Providers in Africa: Review of the Evidence with a Focus on Magnitude, Reach, Cost, and Satisfaction," in *The Lancet* 386 (2015): 1765–1775.
7 John Blevins, Mimi Kiser, Emily Lemon, and Ahoua Kone, "The Percentage of HIV Treatment and Prevention Services in Kenya Provided by Faith-Based Health Providers," in *Development in Practice* 27, no. 5 (2017): 646–657.
8 Joint Learning Initiative on Faith and Local Communities, *Religion and Sustainable Development: Partnerships to End Extreme Poverty. Conference Proceedings* (Washington, DC: Joint Learning Initiative on Faith and Local Communities, 2015), p. 27. Online: https://jliflc.com/wp/wp-content/uploads/2015/08/RSD-Conference-Proceedings_Final.pdf
9 For further information on the ways that PEPFAR and the Global Fund focus on faith-based partnerships, see the following three reports. 1) The U.S. President's Emergency Plan for AIDS Relief, *A Firm Foundation: The PEPFAR Consultation on the Role of Faith-based Organizations in Sustaining Community and Country Leadership in the Response to HIV/AIDS* (Washington, DC: U.S. Department of State, 2012). Online: www.pepfar.gov/documents/organization/195614.pdf 2) The U.S. President's Emergency Plan for AIDS Relief, *Building on Firm Foundations: The PEPFAR Consultation on the Role of Faith-based Organizations in Sustaining Community and Country Leadership in the Response to HIV/AIDS* (Washington, DC: U.S. Department of State, 2015). Online: www.pepfar.gov/documents/organization/247613.pdf and 3) Friends of the Global Fight Against AIDS, Tuberculosis, and Malaria. *A Critical Partnership: The Lifesaving Collaboration Between The Global Fund and Faith-Based Organizations*. Washington, DC: Friends of the Global Fight Against AIDS, Tuberculosis, and Malaria, 2015.
10 United Nations Development Programme. *UNDP Guidelines on Engaging with Faith-Based Organizations and Religious Leaders*. Geneva: United Nations Development Programme, 2014.
11 United Nations Joint Programme on HIV/AIDS. *Partnership with Faith-Based Organizations: UNAIDS Strategic Framework*. Geneva: United Nations Joint Programme on HIV/AIDS, 2009. Online: http://data.unaids.org/pub/report/2010/jc1786_fbo_en.pdf
12 World Health Organization. *Building From Common Foundations: The World Health Organization and Faith-Based Organizations in Primary Healthcare*. Geneva: World Health Organization, 2009. African Religious Health Assets Programme. *Appreciating Assets: The Contribution of Religion to Universal Access in Africa, Report for the World Health Organization*. Cape Town: African Religious Health Assets Programme, 2006. Online: www.irhap.uct.ac.za/sites/default/files/image_tool/images/244/Report_ARHAPWHO_web.pdf
13 UNICEF. *Partnering with Religious Communities for Children*. Geneva: United Nations Children's Fund, 2012. Online: www.unicef.org/eapro/Partnering_with_Religious_Communities_for_Children.pdf
14 Andre Siegfried, *America Comes of Age: A French Analysis* (New York: Harcourt, Brace, and Company, 1927), 33.
15 Michael Barnett and Janice Gross Stein, eds. *Sacred Aid: Faith and Humanitarianism* (New York: Oxford University Press, 2012).
16 Susan R. Holman, *Beholden: Religion, Global Health, and Human Rights* (New York: Oxford University Press, 2015).
17 Gary Gunderson and James Cochrane, *Religion and the Health of the Public: Shifting the Paradigm* (Palgrave MacMillan, 2012).
18 Pamela Klassen, *Spirits of Protestantism: Medicine, Healing and Liberal Christianity* (Berkeley, CA: University of California Press, 2014).
19 See www.thelancet.com/series/faith-based-health-care
20 See www.tandfonline.com/toc/cdip20/27/5?nav=tocList%29
21 Ellen Idler, ed. *Religion as a Social Determinant of Public Health* (New York: Oxford University Press, 2014).
22 Helen Epstein, *The Invisible Cure: Why We Are Losing the Fight Against AIDS in Africa* (New York: Picador, 2008).
23 Scott Evertz, *How Ideology Trumped Science: Why PEPFAR Has Failed to Meet Its Potential* (Washington, DC: Center for American Progress, 2010).

24 Amy E. Black, Douglas L. Koopman, and David K. Ryden, *Of Little Faith: The Politics of George W. Bush's Faith-Based Initiatives* (Washington, DC: Georgetown University Press, 2004).

25 See Blevins, et. al.

References

Barnett, Michael and Janice Gross Stein, eds. *Sacred Aid: Faith and Humanitarianism*. New York: Oxford University Press, 2012.

Black, Amy E., Douglas L. Koopman, and David K. Ryden. *Of Little Faith: The Politics of George W. Bush's Faith-Based Initiatives*. Washington, DC: Georgetown University Press, 2004.

Blevins, John, Mimi Kiser, Emily Lemon, and Ahoua Kone. "The Percentage of HIV Treatment and Prevention Services in Kenya Provided by Faith-Based Health Providers." *Development in Practice* 27, no. 5 (2017): 646–657.

Emmons, Nathanael. *A Sermon, Preached on the Annual Thanksgiving in Massachusetts. November 27, 1800*. Wrentham, MA: Nathaniel Heaton, 1801.

Epstein, Helen. *The Invisible Cure: Why We Are Losing the Fight Against AIDS in Africa*. New York: Picador, 2008.

Evertz, Scott. *How Ideology Trumped Science: Why PEPFAR Has Failed to Meet Its Potential*. Washington, DC: Center for American Progress, 2010.

Good, Charles M. "Pioneer Medical Missions in Africa." *Social Science and Medicine* 32, no. 1 (1991): 1–10.

Gunderson, Gary and James Cochrane. *Religion and the Health of the Public: Shifting the Paradigm*. New York: Palgrave MacMillan, 2012.

Holman, Susan R. *Beholden: Religion, Global Health, and Human Rights*. New York: Oxford University Press, 2015.

Idler, Ellen, ed. *Religion as a Social Determinant of Public Health*. New York: Oxford University Press, 2014.

Joint Learning Initiative on Faith and Local Communities, *Religion and Sustainable Development: Partnerships to End Extreme Poverty. Conference Proceedings*. Washington, DC: Joint Learning Initiative on Faith and Local Communities, 2015.

Klassen, Pamela. *Spirits of Protestantism: Medicine, Healing and Liberal Christianity*. Berkeley, CA: University of California Press, 2014.

Olivier, Jill, Clarence Tsimpo, Regina Gemignani, Mari Shojo, Harold Coulombe, et al. "Understanding the Roles of Faith-Based Health-Care Providers in Africa: Review of the Evidence with a Focus on Magnitude, Reach, Cost, and Satisfaction." *The Lancet* 386 (2015): 1765–1775.

Siegfried, Andre. *America Comes of Age: A French Analysis*. New York: Harcourt, Brace, and Company, 1927.

Worboys, Michael. "The Colonial World as Mission and Mandate." *Osiris* 15 (2000): 207–218.

1 The religious origins of America's relationship to the world

The providence of God, the founding of a nation, and a mission to the world: America's religious roots

On March 22, 1638, Mrs. Anne Hutchinson was excommunicated from her Puritan congregation and expelled from the Massachusetts Bay Colony. Raised as an Anglican in England, Hutchinson followed the Reverend John Cotton to America after Cotton was forced to leave England due to his Puritan beliefs. While her personal life and religious practice were marked by strong faith and devotion, Anne Hutchinson was also a skilled nurse midwife and key health provider to the young colony. Her brother-in-law, the Reverend John Wheelwright, heaped praise on her nursing skills and her compassion:

> Mrs. Anne Hutchinson was a woman of remarkable force of character, intellectual power, and acquirements, as well as of unaffected piety. As a nurse of the sick, especially in the ailments peculiar to her sex, she was singularly skillful, and cheerfully rendered gratuitous service to all who were in need; so that in the infant settlement, where few means of alleviating suffering were to be found, it is not strange that she came to be esteemed as little less than a ministering angel.[1]

Anne Hutchinson was also strong-willed and possessed a keen intellect, traits which did not bode well for a woman in the American colonies in the mid-seventeenth century. She was tried in the civil court of the Massachusetts Bay Colony and found guilty of heresy for her interpretations of the Biblical texts, especially in relation to the nature of God's grace. As evidence of God's wrath for her wrong thinking, prosecutors in the trial cited the malformed stillbirths experienced both by Hutchinson and her husband and by some families who had the misfortune to seek her medical expertise during labor.[2]

The Reverend John Eliot was one of the judges in Hutchinson's trial. Eliot was a Puritan pastor who had immigrated to the Massachusetts from England. Eliot's wife, Ann, was also a medical provider and herbalist in the colony.[3] However, Ann Eliot seemed less inclined to question religious teachings; she was not accused of heresy, tried, and convicted as Anne Hutchinson was. Like his wife, Eliot valued medicine and health care, but neither of these trumped religious faith; the teachings of Puritanism and its call to follow Christ took precedence.

In the years following the Hutchinson trial, Eliot became a missionary to the Native Americans who inhabited the Massachusetts Bay Colony. He learned the Algonquin language and subsequently produced an Algonquin language translation of the Bible. Preaching in the Algonquin tongue, Eliot converted the first groups of Native Americans to the Christian faith in the early 1640s. In his sermon to the Native American leader Waban and his family in 1646, Eliot preached these words:

> Jesus said they that be whole need not a physician, but they that are sick . . . These words are a similitude; that, as some be sick and some well; and we see in experience, that when we be sick, we need a Physician, and go to him and make use of his physic; but they that be well need not do so, they need it not and care not for it; so it is with soul sickness. And we are all sick of that sickness in our souls, but we know it not. We have many at this time, sick in body; for which cause we do fast and pray this day, and cry to God, but more are sick in their souls . . . Therefore, what should we do this day, but go to Christ, the Physician of souls? He healed men's bodies; but he can heal souls also. He is a great Physician; therefore, let all sinners go to him . . . Such as see their sins and are sick of sin, them Christ calleth to repentance and to believe in Christ; therefore, let us see our need of Christ to heal all our disease of soul and body.[4]

While one might assume that Reverend Eliot's tenacity in learning the Algonquin language and eloquence in delivering these words might have had an effect on the conversion of Waban and his family, the illnesses and widespread death among the Algonquin and of other Native American tribes from smallpox and other infections undoubtedly played a role. Numerous Native American settlements had been decimated by infections introduced by the English to which they had no immunity. Estimates of mortality in the years following the first arrival of the English settlers ranged up to 90% among the Pequots, Pawtuxets, and Pokanokets,[5] a devastation described by Neal Salisbury, a historian of Native American cultures, as "a vast disaster zone, comparable to those left by modern wars and other large-scale catastrophes."[6] Under such circumstances, John Eliot's description that "some be sick and some well; and we see in experience that when we be sick, we need a Physician" likely held a rhetorical weight they would not have had not the Native Americans been defeated in battle and decimated by disease.

For Eliot and the Puritan faithful, conversion entailed not only an assent to the tenets of the Christian faith; it required a new way of living. One of Eliot's first reports detailing the work of the Puritans in the American colonies to their brethren back in England described their early efforts to convert Native Americans to Christianity. The report, published in 1643 and entitled *New England's First Fruits; In Respect, First of the Conversion of Some, Conviction of Divers, Preparation of Sundry of the Indians*, details the first conversion of a leader of a Native American tribe. That leader of the Pequot, named Wequash, was exhorted to forsake his wives, his family, and his tribe in his conversion to Christianity. Filled with fear at the power of the Puritans' God who had equipped them to so easily defeat the Pequot, Wequash converted not only to a new religion but a new culture. As a Christian, he lived among the Puritans. The report recounts the death of Wequash. As he lay on his deathbed, some Pequot who had come to visit Wequash exhorted him to go to the *Wigwam*, the healer of the Pequot people. Again, according to the report, Wequash refused, saying "If Jesus Christ say that Wequash shall live, then Wequash must live; if Jesus Christ say, that Wequash shall dye, then Wequash is willing to dye, and will not lengthen out his life by any such meanes."[7]

John Eliot went on to help organize Native American converts to Christianity into "Praying Indian" communities: 14 localities across the colony with the same types governmental and civic institutions—including schools and medical facilities—found in British and American colonial towns. Like Wequash, the Native Americans who professed the Christian faith had to forsake their families and cultures and its spiritual beliefs and institutions. In return, they enjoyed greater trade with the European colonists, had access to better land, and received education and health care provided by the British settlers that they prayed would save them from an all-too-common death.[8]

The histories of John Eliot and Anne Hutchinson demonstrate the connections between religion and health. Eliot offered testimony to God's Providential care of their community as well as their role in ensuring the salvation of the Native Americans. For the Puritans, such testimony never considered the cost of conversion to the Native Americans themselves or to the violence of conquest of the land, either through armed conflict or the introduction of disease. For the pious Puritans looking to understand the relationship between their faith in God and health, Hutchinson served as an object lesson that misguided beliefs expressed in her heretical perspectives on the nature of God's grace—perspectives expressed as a woman, no less—would incur God's wrath which took the form of miscarriages and malformed infants. For these Protestant Christians who were among the first Europeans to settle in the New World, religious beliefs and practices were entwined with conceptions of health and illness, not only in their own communities, but also (even especially) in their mission activities to the Native Americans they encountered.

Eliot was not the only person involved in Protestant missionary efforts to the Native Americans. By no means did they all share the same attitude toward Native Americans culture as the one reflected in the description of Wequash's renouncement of his family and culture. The Moravians, following the expectation of their European benefactor Count Nicolaus Zinzendorf, made no demands on Native

Americans to leave their families, communities, or cultures behind. The Moravians believed any mission work should be short-term and geared toward equipping the people to whom the work was focused to take on the structures for Christian worship and nurture according to their own cultural context.[9] Quaker missionaries assumed that Indian culture revealed "the Inner Light" which could not be limited only to the structures of European civilization to be grasped. Quaker missionary John Woolman saw Indian culture as a resource for his own learning and a source for revelation claiming

> I was inwardly joyful that the Lord had strengthened me to come on this [missionary] visit [to the Indians], and had manifested a fatherly care over me in my poor lowly condition, when, in my own eyes, I appeared inferior to many among the Indians.[10]

The Baptist missionary Roger Williams dissented from the approach of the Praying Indian communities, seeing his call to be a missionary *among* the Indian and not *to* them. Williams believed that conversion was not a matter of intellectual assent but a conviction that the Christian religion offered Native Americans a way to better live a life marked by love and humility.[11] This position stood in sharp contrast to that of Cotton Mather, an influential Puritan leader not only in Massachusetts but across the American colonies, who regarded the spiritual practices of Native Americans as a form of devil-worship and wrote that it would be "the most unexceptionable piece of justice in the world for to extinguish the offending savages."[12]

Given these widely varying attitudes, it is little wonder Native Americans themselves were confused and wary. David Brainerd, a Presbyterian missionary to Native Americans in the mid-eighteenth century, recounted an exchange with Native Americans that demonstrates this confusion and wariness:

> [The Indians] asked me why I desired the Indians to become *Christians*, seeing the Christians were so much worse than the Indians and were more adept at lying, stealing, and drinking, I assured them that the whites they referred to were the bad whites. I and the ones who sent me, I explained, were the good whites who would never steal Indian land. The Indians then asked, plaintively, why did not these good people send you to teach us before, while we had our lands down by the seaside? . . . [Their decision to become Christians] was a favour they could not now be so good as to shew me, seeing they had received so many injuries from the *white* people.[13]

The missionary programs established by various Protestant groups in the American colonies to the Native Americans whose home was the land these Europeans Christians claimed as their own are an early example of Protestant foreign missions. In this instance, however, they are examples of foreign missions undertaken by English Protestants, not American. That those mission enterprises were carried out hand-in-hand with the practices of colonization should surprise no one and this marriage between religion and empire will be a familiar trope in this book. The English Puritans, Presbyterians, Baptists, and other Protestants who traveled to America from England beginning in the seventeenth century had no conception of a new nation known as the United States. Their vision was grounded in theological conviction and not in a model of governance. For these early colonial settlers, the societies they were establishing in the American colonies were evidence of God's plan for the redemption of the world. Missionary activities to the Native Americans residing in the colonies provided an additional rationale for their endeavors. In fact, the call to bring the message of the Christian gospel to the Native Americans was a primary driver of the English Puritans' immigration to the American colonies.

In 1629, the charter of the Massachusetts Bay Colony listed a primary reason for the establishment of the colony: "the duty to win and invite the natives of the country to the knowledge of the only true God and Savior."[14] In 1649, the Long Parliament in England granted a charter for the New England Company to carry out business enterprises in the colony for the purpose of raising funds with the stipulation that they support the evangelization of the Native Americans.[15] The "Praying Indian" communities that Eliot helped establish were a model of governance not only for the Native Americans tribes to whom he preached; Eliot advocated for a similar government structure both for the American colonies and for England.

In his treatise *The Christian Commonwealth: or, The Civil Policy of The Rising Kingdom of Jesus Christ*, Eliot called for a structure of government based upon the model instituted by Moses when he led the Israelites in the wilderness following their release from captivity in Egypt. For Eliot the parallels between those events and the lives of seventeenth-century New Englanders was clear: God had delivered a people chosen to be a light to the world from a tyrannical form of government, and these same chosen people had a sacred duty to implement God's providential intentions for all the world through this new form of government. The Israelites might have been unfaithful to such a call but the Puritans of New England would fulfill that obligation.[16]

Eliot's view was common. In 1630, when John Winthrop led some of the earliest Puritan immigrants to the new colony in America, he preached a sermon on the deck of the *Arabella*, the ship that had carried the group, proclaiming that this group of the faithful were not establishing a wholly new government but perfecting one bequeathed to them by the faithful who had come before. Their efforts to institute God's reign in the governance of other societies was thwarted by corrupt and worldly governments, the most recent example being the British government from whom they had to flee. In establishing a new society in the Massachusetts colony, these Puritans had an opportunity—an obligation—to institute a government based on Christian principles taught them by the faithful in England whose example served as the foundation for the new world.

> Whatsoever we did, or ought to have done, when we lived in England, the same must we do, and more also, where we go. That which the most in their churches maintain as truth in profession only, we must bring into familiar and constant practice; as in this duty of love, we must love brotherly without dissimulation, we must love one another with a pure heart fervently. We must bear one another's burdens.[17]

In this same sermon, Winthrop famously described this new colony as a city upon a hill:

> For we must consider that we shall be as a city upon a hill. The eyes of all people are upon us. So that if we shall deal falsely with our God in this work we have undertaken, and so cause Him to withdraw His present help from us, we shall be made a story and a by-word through the world . . . [I] shut this discourse with that exhortation of Moses, that faithful servant of the Lord, in his last farewell to Israel, Deut. 30. "Beloved, there is now set before us life and death, good and evil," in that we are commanded this day to love the Lord our God, and to love one another, to walk in his ways and to keep his Commandments and his ordinance and his laws, and the articles of our Covenant with Him, that we may live and be multiplied, and that the Lord our God may bless us in the land whither we go to possess it. But if our hearts shall turn away, so that we will not obey, but shall be seduced, and worship other Gods, our pleasure and profits, and serve them; it is propounded unto us this day, we shall surely perish out of the good land whither we pass over this vast sea to possess it. Therefore, let us choose life, that we and our seed may live, by obeying His voice and cleaving to Him, for He is our life and our prosperity.[18]

As the first governor of the Massachusetts colony, Winthrop worked tirelessly to establish a government built on the model of Christian community he so fervently sought to emulate. Of course, such efforts would be difficult to maintain in the face of disagreements about what exactly constituted such Christian communities. In 1648, the Puritan congregations in the colony ratified the Cambridge Platform spelling out their positions on questions of doctrine and polity. In the coming decades these positions became the legal standard, not only for the Massachusetts colony but in similar ways for the Connecticut colony, which established a more formal relationship between church doctrine and the laws of the colony through the Saybrook Articles of 1708.[19]

These Protestant leaders in the American colonies were united in their belief that America had a specific destiny in helping to bring about God's kingdom on earth. In his treatise, *Magnalia Christi Americani*, Cotton Mather argued that God's mission for the salvation of the world was linked to America's destiny.[20] Jonathan Edwards, the Puritan pastor whose sermons helped set the spark for the religious revival in America known as the Great Awakening, believed that America was the site from which God's final work of the redemption of the world prior to the return of Christ had begun.[21]

Various historians have noted the significance of this Puritan belief in America's distinctive and essential role in God's plan for humanity. The American historian Walter McDougall argued that American principles had their antecedent in the European societies from which the colonists came and that those principles could only come to full flower in the colony: "In the eyes of the Founding Fathers, clergymen, publicists, and other opinion leaders the new nation was a distillation of virtues *latent* in the civilization they left behind, but susceptible of realization only in America."[22] Likewise, the religious historian William Hutchison described the belief in America's role as God's instrument put forth by Puritan leaders this way:

> America . . . was not the realm of outer darkness into which, in the parable, the unworthy servant is cast. Though haughty European theologians had thought otherwise, America was a region . . . where the saving light of the Gospel had come to shine, and where "true and original Christianity" was flourishing. It was the land where, beyond all others, essential Christianity could be practiced and propagated—removed as the New World was from the sectarian faction of the Old. America, besides being the continent where many of the heathens had been sequestered, was a place where one could recover the very Gospel that must be preached to them: the simple Christian message, the *evangelium aeternam*.[23]

Theologically, the notion of America as God's instrument was tied to the belief in the immanent return of Jesus to earth. The Christian Scriptures speak of the return of Christ to earth to fulfill God's kingdom as the culmination of history, and while various interpretations of this idea have arisen in Christianity over the course of the tradition, American Protestants believed that America was destined to play a key role in hastening that return. The belief in Christ's return was called millennialism in reference to the twentieth chapter of the biblical book of *Revelation*, which speaks of a 1,000-year reign of the kingdom of God that occurs in context with Christ's return. While there were sharp disagreements as to whether the fulfillment of God's reign on earth was a necessary prerequisite to Christ's return (post-millennialism) or whether his return would mark the start of the 1,000-year reign of God on earth (pre-millennialism),[24] either interpretation fueled the zeal for foreign missions. If Christ could only return after God's reign was achieved on earth, then there was no time to waste in assuring that nations who had not yet heard the message of the Christian tradition could hear and receive the good news.

If the return of Christ ushered in God's reign as the forces of evil were swept away, then there was no time to waste in giving "the heathen" a chance to accept Christ before he returned in judgment of all those who had not accepted him. A pamphlet published by the American Board of Commissioners for Foreign Missions (ABCFM) is only one among numerous examples of theological writing from the first decades of the new nation that demonstrate the connections between millennialism and foreign mission:

> I find myself between two worlds; that which we now inhabit and that where sinners redeemed by the grace of the gospel dwell. I look towards this world—and lo! The elements are melting with fervent heat; the earth and all the works therein are on fire: its palaces, its villages, its cities—all its pleasant and magnificent things, are sinking into ruin. I look to the other world, and there I see redeemed men, rising in knowledge, felicity, and glory, till imagination is lost in the beauty and grandeur of the vision.—With these things in view, hasten, all ye friends of missions, hasten, and rescue from the coming conflagration a portion of the wealth of this world, and with it raise multitudes of perishing heathens to that world of light and glory.[25]

American exceptionalism: religion and the politics of the new nation

The Protestants who first arrived in the American colonies in the early 1600s were initially inspired by a *theological* vision of sharing the gospel with the "heathen Indians" and of building a society that anticipated the imminent return of Jesus. Over a century later, however, the realities of this world had begun to crowd out visions of the world to come and while the nation's political motivations might echo these theological narratives, they did not exactly mirror them. While a few political leaders in the colonial period and in the first decades of the new nation may have expressed millennialist perspectives,[26] most emphasized American exceptionalism without reference to Jesus's return. A narrative of that exceptionalism served political purposes.

Discontent toward the British crown, while by no means universal, was growing and the various colonies had begun to develop a system of shared representation in relation to the British crown. Although religious freedom was often invoked as a reason for the colonies' founding and part of their essential character, in its very first official act the Continental Congress lodged a formal protest to the British Parliament upon its passage of the Quebec Act in 1774. Among other matters, the Act granted freedom of worship to Roman Catholics under English rule in the Quebec province of the Canadian colonies.[27] Religious freedom, it seemed, was limited to *Protestant* Christianity alone.

As calls for independence from the British crown grew across the colonies, the earlier theological belief that God had chosen Protestant Christians to bring to fruition the redemption of the world was supplemented by political claims: the new American nation would hold an exceptional role among the world's governments. Many historians have noted the force and resiliency of this idea of American exceptionalism. However, many analyze the development of this idea—at least in regard to America's orientation to the world—in the last half of the nineteenth century. In fact, the new nation included foreign policy as a focus from the beginning and this religious belief played a role. The diplomatic relationship of the colonies to both England and France had decisive effects on the course of the American revolutionary war. French support of the British colonies in America in their fight for independence from the crown provided essential strategic and military power to the colonists. American political leaders, however, carried out a complex set of negotiations between England and France (along with the other European powers who supported the French position), and the terms of the 1783 Paris Treaty ending the war demonstrated the benefits of this non-alliance approach for the new nation; those terms were far more generous in laying out the boundaries of the new nation than any of those fighting independence would have dared hope.

The Articles of Confederation laid out the structure of governance for the new nation. They were written and ratified during the course of the war, but the individual states (the former colonies) in America were wary of the authority of the national government to negotiate treaties with other national governments; questions of foreign policy revealed one of the most striking problems with the first governance structure of the United States. The new nation's leaders gathered to draft a new Constitution, which was completed in 1787. Three of those leaders—Alexander Hamilton, John Jay, and James Madison—published a series of 85 essays over the course of eight months in 1787–1788 in three newspapers in New York advocating for the citizens of New York to ratify the new Constitution. Those complete series of essays came to be known as *The Federalist Papers*, and 29 of those essays focused specifically on the country's relationship to foreign powers.[28]

After the ratification of the Constitution, the United States continued to pursue a policy of independent engagement with both England and France. As the French Revolution unfolded, there was a strong and growing sentiment among many American citizens to break culturally and politically with the British and side with the new democratic republic in France. But the cultural ties to England—particularly the religious connections—were too strong.

At its founding, a key element of America's conception of its own exceptionalism was grounded in the idea that it was perfecting the social, political, and religious structures of Anglo-Saxon England and that it would show to the world the power and moral rightness of those structures through its own government and society.[29] This idea, reflected in the political positions of the nation's leaders, was also held by Protestant Christian leaders. That obligation was not to mold their religious communities or their new nation according to the European societies they had left behind but to perfect the structure of those societies in America, thereby renewing Protestant Europe, especially England. For America's religious leaders, European religious renewal was essential if the church was to be faithful in fulfilling God's plan because Europe provided the economic, military, and political power to take the gospel to the rest of the world. In short, a key element driving the nation's self-understanding of its foreign affairs was a missionary belief that God had called the nation to save the world.[30]

In the half century after the nation's founding, this notion of American responsibility had crystallized into a firm, sustained commitment for the foreign missionary endeavors of American Protestants. From 1789–1828, donations to charitable organizations rivaled the entire outlay of the federal government; while total cumulative expenditures by the U.S. government were approximately 3.6 million dollars, the cumulative revenues of the largest dozen charities in the same time period were 2.8 million dollars. The American Board of Commissioners for Foreign Missions (ABCFM), a body made of Protestant religious leaders representing their respective denominations to support shared mission activities, was the second largest charitable organization in the United States; only the American Education Society was larger. Additionally, the foreign missions agencies of the American Baptist Churches and of the Dutch Reformed Church were eighth and twelfth in size.[31]

During the economic crisis of 1831, some critics raised concerns that the ABCFM was sending so much money abroad that it was de-stabilizing the national economy. In response, advocates for the ABCFM argued that support of foreign missions was "the dew of gospel charity on the moral wilderness [of other countries]." Support of foreign missions, they claimed, had so energized Christians in the United States that it had led to a religious revival across the country.[32] Whatever the causes, statistics on church attendance during this this time reflect a rapid rise in church affiliation. At the dawn of the American revolution in 1776, only 17% of the colonists noted any formal church membership, but by 1850, that number had grown to 34%.[33]

This surge in church affiliation was a direct outgrowth of the religious revival that swept across the country in the 1830s. That religious movement, known today as the Second Great Awakening, also marked a shift in the intellectual forces shaping American Christianity as well as the social sites of its power. The nation's religious mainstream had been centered on European theologies guided by Enlightenment thinking, Anglican church structures and rituals (or the revivalist offshoots of Anglicanism in Britain), and the social and academic institutions of New England. In the days after the War of 1812 against the British,[34] this perspective was echoed by the Boston Puritan minister, Edward Dorr Griffin:

> If the Church, now chiefly confined to two countries [the United States and her current enemy, Great Britain], is to rise from this day forth, where is it more likely to rise than in the United States, the most favored spot on this continent which was discovered, as I may say, by the light of the Reformation!

> And if in the United States, where rather than in New England? And if in New England, where rather than Massachusetts, which has been blessed by the prayers of so long a succession of godly ancestors?[35]

By the middle decades of the nineteenth century, Protestant evangelicalism had changed the country's religious landscape. In 1776, Puritan Congregationalists accounted for 20% of all religious adherents in the American colonies; by 1850, that number was only 4%. During the same period, Methodists grew from just 2.5% to 34% and Baptists from 2% to 22%; each was influenced by evangelical religious practice and belief.[36] Marked by emotional fervor, social critique, and millennialist theology, evangelicalism provided an impetus both for progressive social movements such as abolition, temperance, and suffrage and ushered in sharp debates about theological doctrines. In the coming decades, these forces would eventually lead to sharp divides within Protestantism on both social-political and theological grounds.[37]

As America headed into the middle decades of the nineteenth century emboldened by a victory over the British in the War of 1812, political leaders began to implement the notion of American exceptionalism in two ways: first, as a context for articulating the nation's position on colonization in North America in what came to be known as the Monroe Doctrine; and second, as a basis for expansionism across the continent. In his State of the Union address to the US Congress in 1823, President Monroe referenced wars currently being fought among European powers and expressed the nation's non-interventionist stance in regard to those conflicts. He then set forth the nation's position against the imposition of those nations into the interests of the United States. While noting the good diplomatic relations that the United States enjoyed with the European powers, Monroe also claimed that

> we owe it, therefore, to candor and to the amicable relations existing between the United States and those powers to declare that we should consider any attempt on their part to extend their system to any portion of this hemisphere as dangerous to our peace and safety. With the existing colonies or dependencies of any European power we have not interfered and shall not interfere . . . It is impossible that the allied powers [of Europe] should extend their political system to any portion of either continent without endangering our peace and happiness; nor can anyone believe that our southern brethren, if left to themselves, would adopt it of their own accord. It is equally impossible, therefore, that we should behold such interposition in any form with indifference.[38]

The position articulated in the speech came to be known as the Monroe Doctrine; it became a cornerstone for American foreign policy and would figure directly into the nation's decision to go to war with Spain at the end of the nineteenth century, as we shall see. In 1823, however, the position was a political articulation of the religious idea of American exceptionalism because it articulated the distinction between the nation and the European powers to which it was most closely allied. America would chart a different course, and while it would respect the sovereignty of those European powers, the country's leaders were nonetheless clear that the sovereignty of the United States would also be respected.

In regard to the second issue, the relationship between exceptionalism and expansionism, Americans believed that God had given to this nation a distinctive role in history and had blessed the country with a rich and expansive land which it must claim in order to transfer the empire of the world. During the War of 1812, William Henry Harrison, then governor of the territory of Indiana (the territory would become a state a few years later in 1816), claimed,

> Is one of the fairest portions of the globe to remain in a state of nature, the haunt of a few wretched savages, when it seems destined by the Creator to give support to a large population and to be the seat of civilization, of science, and of true religion?[39]

Arguments such as Harrison's would grow as the nation pushed into the frontier territories of its Western borders.[40] Both the War Department of the federal government and the foreign missions bodies of Protestant denominations saw these frontier lands as foreign. Though it supported extensive mission enterprises in China, India, and the Sandwich Islands (known today as the state of Hawaii), the ABCFM sent about 20% of its missionaries to evangelize Native Americans. The missionary impulse of British Protestants to evangelize the New World as a foreign missions endeavor had transferred to the first generations of American Protestants who continued to view Native Americans as foreign heathen to be converted and not as the pre-existing inhabitants of the land that these Christians had claimed as their own. Such missions endeavors entered into the "foreign lands" of the Native Americans hand-in-hand with the aspirations of the nation's political leaders.[41]

America's belief that it was destined to be a unique instrument for God in the salvation of the world was cultivated in the religious heritage of British Protestantism, the theological beliefs of Millennialism, and the expansionist impulses of its political leaders. In 1845, these viewpoints were fully spelled out by the newspaper columnist John O'Sullivan in an article in *The United States Democratic Review* entitled "The Great Nation of Futurity":

> Our national birth was the beginning of a new history, the formation and progress of an untried political system, which separates us from the past and connects us with the future only; and so far as regards the entire development of the natural rights of man, in moral, political, and national life, we may confidently assume that our country is destined to be the great nation of futurity.

> America is destined for better deeds . . . The expansive future is our arena, and for our history. We are entering on its untrodden space, with the truths of God in our minds, beneficent objects in our hearts, and with a clear conscience unsullied by the past. We are the nation of human progress, and who will, what can, set limits to our onward march? . . .
>
> The far-reaching, the boundless future will be the era of American greatness. In its magnificent domain of space and time, the nation of many nations is *destined* to *manifest* to mankind the excellence of divine principles; to establish on earth the noblest temple ever dedicated to the worship of the Most High—the Sacred and the True . . . This is our high destiny, and in nature's eternal, inevitable decree of cause and effect we must accomplish it. All this will be our future history, to establish on earth the moral dignity and salvation of man—the immutable truth and beneficence of God. For this blessed mission to the nations of the world, which are shut out from the life-giving light of truth, has America been chosen; and her high example shall smite unto death the tyranny of kings, hierarchs, and oligarchs, and carry the glad tidings of peace and good will where myriads now endure an existence scarcely more enviable than that of beasts of the field. Who, then, can doubt that our country is destined to be the great nation of futurity?[42]

O'Sullivan was the first to refer to a *manifest destiny* of the nation, but the term endured and today refers to the common belief in the nation at the time that America not only had a right but an obligation to expand in order to birth a new form of government and a new society which all other nations would emulate, in keeping with the will of God.

America's westward expansion was incessant. This expansion necessitated the forced, often violent displacement of Native Americans and negotiations with foreign governments[43] but Americans were certain of their divine right to make those lands from the country's Western border to the Pacific Ocean part of their nation. A theological notion of Divine Providence had merged with political power and national aspiration to create the idea that expansion was America's manifest destiny. In the latter decades of the nineteenth century, that idea would grow to influence the nation's understanding of its interests around the globe.

A mission of health: mission and public health practice in these new United States

Up to this point, this book has provided a historical summary of the questions of America's relationship to the rest of the world from religious and political perspectives. Influences from public health and development practice have not been part of this narrative because they were not established fields of research or practice in the time period examined so far. There are, however, some political and scientific events in this time that are important to note for their role in setting the stage for the addition of public health and development practice to this history in the coming decades.

The mid-1700s marked the first large-scale efforts at vaccination in America. Although the germ theory of disease had not yet been developed, there were efforts to confer immunization from infection through a controlled exposure to that infection. The idea of inoculation through a scratch of an instrument that had been exposed to the contagion was controversial. A smallpox epidemic in the Massachusetts colony in 1721 had led the Puritan minister Cotton Mather to call for inoculation of the (British) inhabitants of the colony. His advocacy was not always well received. In November of that year, an anonymous protester threw a small bomb into Mather's home. The bomb did not detonate, but the intent was clear—attached to the device was the following message: "Cotton Mather, you dog, dam you! I'll inoculate you with this; with a pox to you."[44]

In 1776, the Continental Army forbade its surgeons from carrying out inoculations,[45] but when smallpox broke out among Canadian soldiers fighting in Quebec that year, the American forces decided that inoculation was required. Ninety percent of all deaths among these soldiers was due to illness, with smallpox being the chief culprit. General George Washington ordered the inoculation of the entire Continental Army in 1777,[46] despite controversies over the dangers of inoculation. Smallpox inoculation would not be improved upon for another 20 years, but in 1798, Edward Jenner discovered a vaccine to confer immunity to smallpox could be produced from cowpox, a far less virulent virus for humans.[47]

In that same year, the U.S. Congress passed and President Adams signed *An Act for the Relief of Sick and Disabled Seamen*. The importance of a strong shipping economy, the relationship of this economy to the nation's political and military self-interest, and the fear of infection from returning sailors led to the law, which allowed for the collection of a tax from the wages of each sailor with funds raised to provide hospitals for those sailors. These hospitals, located at the nation's major ports, provided a first line of defense against potential contagions being brought to the country by returning ships, as well as one of the first organizational structures in the nation to provide ongoing, sustained medical care to a particular group. In time, the organizational structure initiated through these facilities would become the U.S. Public Health Service.[48] In 1797, just one year prior to the passage of this new law and the discovery of cowpox, the nation's first medical journal, *The Medical Repository*, began publication. By 1850, the number of medical journals published in the United States would top 250.[49]

The War of 1812 would mark not only a shift in America's relationship to England, it was also the period in which the U.S. Congress established the Office of the Physician and Surgeon General;[50] in time, this office would come to manage the U.S. Public Health Service. In 1831, a cholera epidemic spread across many parts of the globe, with a significant factor in the spread of the infection attributed to

Muslims traveling to Mecca for the hajj, the annual pilgrimage that is a central tenet of Islam. An estimated 20,000 were infected, or 40% of all who made the pilgrimage that year.[51] The epidemic spread globally over the next year and by June 1832, health officials in Toronto and Montreal were announcing over 400 new cases every day with a mortality rate of approximately 50%[52] Health officials in Philadelphia traveled to Canada to gain firsthand insight into the epidemic and decided on a drastic measure to wash all city streets daily with steamed water. The city published information on the spread of the disease and on measures to prevent that spread in a series of 16 papers called *The Cholera Gazette*. The epidemic was slowed but not halted and scores were infected in the city. Nonetheless, in a final analysis on the factors that contributed to fewer infections and lower rates of mortality, those same officials concluded that

> a well-regulated sanitary police, and public measures of hygienic character, having in view the preservation of cleanliness, the prevention of a crowded population, and the procurement of free ventilation are the most efficient means of guarding the community against a very extensive and destructive prevalence of the disease.[53]

That analysis demonstrates both a public health approach to the outbreak and the mistaken theory of "bad air" (miasma theory) for the cause of disease. It would be another 20 years before another cholera epidemic (this time in London in 1854) was halted by identifying that the infection was spread not through foul or stale air but by a water source infected with feces. The outbreak was halted when a physician named John Snow removed the handle from a water pump from which the contaminated water was drawn; the assistance of the local Anglican Parish priest, Henry Whitehead, was essential in Snow's efforts to trace the source of the outbreak—a clear example of a synergy between religion and health. The effort to identify to identify a correlation between infections and the use of the pump is often seen as the birth of modern epidemiology.[54]

Advances in medical knowledge were transforming the practice of medicine to include measures to address population-level health. These examples represent early instances of public health as it is understood today, even if there was no concept of this field of research and practice at the time. The medical advances that allowed such new practices also had an impact on the practice of foreign missions. For a number of years, missionaries and religious leaders had debated the primary purpose of missions and the means by which that purpose would be achieved. Were missions primarily focused on the conversion of "heathens" to the Christian faith, or was their proper focus responding to the needs of others? Were foreign missions only concerned with bringing the gospel to far-flung lands, or was part of their purpose to initiate the cultural and political structures of America in these new nations?

Up through the mid-nineteenth century, such debates often centered on whether missions should also include efforts to "civilize the heathen" to whom the gospel was brought by replicating American institutions. The civilizing influence of missions was often understood in relation to educational institutions or efforts at economic development (for example, in teaching a trade).

Health care was a different matter. Through the colonial era and for the first 40 years of the new nation, medical practice was primarily limited to the skillful use of herbs and medicinal remedies, and the hallmark of "sound medical practice" was a well-stocked medicine bag. An account of the clinical treatment of patients in 1813 at the Marine Hospital in Massachusetts (one of the hospitals opened under the 1798 law that laid the foundation for the U.S. Public Health Service) detailed that

> the patients were bled, purged and given emetics. They were prescribed brown mixture, pills, calomel, mineral water, aloes, nitre, opium, ipecac and dozens of other potions. Teas made from various barks were a part of the treatment of every disease of the digestive tract. If there was a place to put a blister on a pain, it was done. And aches were rubbed with volatile liniment.[55]

The care offered by medical professionals in America's hospitals was not significantly different from that provided by herbalists, traditional healers, or itinerant Methodist pastors.[56] With the medical advances that came at a dizzying pace in the nineteenth century, medicine became an instrument for missionary endeavors. In 1845, Rufus Anderson, senior secretary of the ABCFM, argued that medical services were essential and that they must be offered because the Christian faith demanded care for those in need. They could not be conditional upon confession of faith. Medical care was not, for him, something to be subsumed under the civilizing influence of the missionary relation or as a strategy for achieving the primary end of conversion; rather, medical care was a legitimate end of the foreign missions endeavor because the Christian faith demanded care for the sick.[57]

From this perspective, then, it is hardly surprising to see that the expansionist interests of the United States, the nascent public health initiatives of the Marine Hospitals, and the foreign missions fervor of American Protestants coalesced in the Sandwich Islands. The British had established a presence in the Islands as early as the late 1700s, but by the mid-nineteenth century, the United States began to see a strategic interest in establishing its own presence in these Pacific islands to guard trade routes and safeguard its own western borders. In 1837, a Marine Hospital was established to provide medical care to seamen and ensure that they did not bring infections back to the mainland United States with them. The ABCFM sent the first medical missionaries to the islands in 1842, and those missionary doctors served in rotation to both the mission and the government facilities. Evangelism, health care, and political interests aligned. By the beginning of the twentieth century, the islands were a territory of the United States and today are known as the state of Hawaii.[58]

By the middle of the nineteenth century, the United States was charting a course through the social and political changes that were beginning to shape the modern world. Global politics were in upheaval, as many European nations saw the collapse or restructuring of their respective monarchies even as rise in technological, economic, and military powers drove colonization. The medical advances of the period—a few of which were briefly named above—would usher in a new era of medical care grounded in science. Driven in large part by technological advances, large-scale industries emerged for the first time, and capitalist economic systems began to emerge. Calls for social reform grew louder, even as resistance to changing old ways remained; it would be another half century before many of those initial calls bore fruit in structural change.

Scientific advances were leading to fundamental changes in medical practice and the academic study of the Christian religion experienced fundamental changes as well. Historical-critical methods of interpreting biblical texts in light of their historical and cultural contexts led to crises of meaning about the nature of divine revelation. The dominance of theological studies in European and North American universities began to be challenged, and the question of the relationship between faith and reason became a subject of debate, especially in the colleges and universities founded and funded by religious bodies. Acrimonious debates on both these theological questions and social concerns created further tensions on the fault lines that existed between Evangelical and mainline Protestants. But by the middle of the nineteenth century, the question of slavery in the United States had emerged as the defining issue that eventually led to schisms across various Protestant bodies.

Support for abolition of slavery in the United States had been growing since the eighteenth century, as had a growing, entrenched resistance to abolition. Protestant pastors were key leaders on both sides of the issue. The abolitionist effort with the closest connection to Protestant foreign missions was the American Colonization Society (ACS). Founded in 1816 by the Reverend Robert Finney, the ACS sought to create a movement in which freed black men and women in the United States would live in colonies established in western Africa. The ACS established a colony on the Pepper Colony in 1822, which became the nation of Liberia in 1848. Many of the strongest supporters of the ACS saw the efforts of manumission and resettlement back on African lands as an expression of Protestant foreign mission and the ACS worked with the ABCFM to send freed black men and women as missionaries to Western Africa to minister to the ACS colonies.

No clear consensus about the effectiveness of ACS exists or even whether the organization actually supported abolition or the cause of slavery. Because freed black men and women were offered the chance to leave the United States to return to West Africa, slave owners supported the organization because they believed that the presence of freed black women and men in their communities would contribute to anger and eventual rebellion among those who remained enslaved. The religious leaders who supported ACS were by and large vocal critics of slavery, but the approach of establishing colonies of former slaves in West Africa was disruptive to the existing cultures in those lands, dismissive of the rights of freed black women and men born in the United States, and was used politically by supporters of slavery to disrupt and break apart communities of former slaves.[59]

Disagreements about the motivations and the impact of the ACS should come as no surprise. Slavery was a violent, dehumanizing social institution in the United States and its effects have reverberated throughout the country for centuries. The Protestant denominations would not, by and large, remain intact but would instead split over the slavery issue. Some bodies, such as the Society of Friends (or Quakers) were unified in their abolitionist position, but most denominations split across the geographical divide of the northern and southern states—a geographic boundary that also marked a culture divide. In 1844, Methodists split into two separate bodies. The Baptists followed in 1845. Tensions among Presbyterians over theological differences had led to a split in 1837 into Old School and New School Presbyterians. Both of those bodies split along geographical lines over slavery and by 1864, the two groups in the north had reunited, and the two groups in the south had reunited. Theological differences, it seemed, might be bridged, but positions on slavery and race sustained the divide.[60] In the years after the Civil War, divergent theological positions and social views would harden the dividing lines of American Protestantism; these different expressions of Christianity would each have different relationships to and influences on America's global health and social development programs moving forward.

Notes

1 Charles Bell, "Memoir of John Wheelwright," in *John Wheelwright: His Writings, Including His Fast Day Sermon 1637 and his Mercurius Americanus, 1645;With a Paper on the Genuineness of the Indian Deed of 1629* (Boston: The Prince Society, 1876), 7.

2 See Lindal Buchanan, "A Study of Maternal Rhetoric: Anne Hutchinson, Monsters, and the Antinomian Controversy," in *Rhetoric Review* 25, no. 3 (2009): 239–259.

3 See Patricia Watson, "The 'Hidden Ones': Women and Healing in Colonial New England," in *Medicine and Health*, Peter Burns, ed. (Boston: Boston University Press, 1992), 26.

4 Martin Moore, *Memoirs of the Life and Character of Rev. John Eliot, Apostle of the N.A. Indians* (Boston: Flagg & Gould, 1822), 79–80.

5 Julius H. Rubin, *Tears of Repentance: Christian Indian Identity and Community in Colonial Southern New England* (Lincoln, NE: University of Nebraska Press, 2013), 21. Rubin is quoting mortality rates from Alfred Crosby, *Ecological Imperialism: The Biological Expansion of Europe, 900–1900* (Cambridge: Cambridge University Press, 1986), 284–285 and David E. Stannard, *American Holocaust: The Conquest of the New World* (New York: Oxford University Press, 1992), 108–109.

6 Neal Salisbury, *Manitou and Providence: Indians, Europeans, and the Making of New England, 1500–1643* (New York: Oxford University Press, 1982), 103.

7 John Eliot, *New England's First Fruits; In Respect, First of the Conversion of Some, Conviction of Divers, Preparation of Sundry of the Indians* (London: Henry Overton, 1643), 15.

8 William R. Hutchison, *Errand to the World: American Protestant Thought and Foreign Missions* (Chicago: University of Chicago Press, 1987), 27.

9 Ibid., p. 26.
10 Ibid., pp. 32–33.
11 Ibid., pp. 36–37.
12 Ibid., pp. 38–39.
13 Ibid., p. 31.
14 Ibid., p. 24.
15 Wilbert R. Shenk, "Introduction," in *North American Foreign Missions, 1810–1914*, William R. Shenk, ed. (Grand Rapids, MI: Eerdmans Publishing, 2004), 2.
16 John Eliot, *The Christian Commonwealth: Or, The Civil Policy Of The Rising Kingdom of Jesus Christ* (London: Liverwell Chapman, 1659).
17 See John Winthrop, "A Model of Christian Charity," in *The Journals of John Winthrop*, Richard S. Dunn and Laetitia Yeandle, eds. (Cambridge, MA: The Belknap Press of Harvard University Press, 1996), 8–9.
18 Ibid., p. 12.
19 See Wendy J. Deichman Edwards, "Forging an Ideology for American Missions: Josiah Strong and Manifest Destiny," in *North American Foreign Missions, 1810–1914*, William R. Shenk, ed. (Grand Rapids, MI: Eerdmans Publishing, 2004), 165. For further information on influence of the Cambridge Platform and Saybrook Articles on the governance of the Massachusetts and Connecticut colonies, see Williston Walker, "Massachusetts and the Saybrook Platform" in *Yale Historical Review* 1, no. 1 (1892): 69–86.
20 See Cotton Mather, *Magnalia Christi Americana or The Ecclesial History of New England, Vols. I and II*, Kenneth B. Murdock, ed. (Cambridge, MA: Belknap Press of Harvard University Press, 1977). For a discussion of Mather's perspectives and their influence on America's self-identity see William R. Hutchison, *Errand to the World: American Protestant Thought and Foreign Missions* (Chicago: University of Chicago Press, 1987) 39–41.
21 Ibid., pp. 41–42.
22 Walter A. McDougall, *Promised Land, Crusader State: The American Encounter with the World Since 1776* (New York: Houghton Mifflin, 1997), 17.
23 Hutchison, pp. 39–40.
24 An in-depth study of different perspectives on millennialism is beyond the scope of this text. What is clear, however, is the central role of millennialist beliefs in the fervor surrounding foreign missions. For more discussion of this role, see Richard Lee Rogers, "A Bright and New Constellation: Millennial Narratives and the Origins of American Foreign Missions," in *North American Foreign Missions, 1810–1914*, William R. Shenk, ed. (Grand Rapids, MI: Eerdmans Publishing, 2004), 39–60. Also, see Hutchison, especially chapter 4.
25 D.T. Kimball and Lyman Beecher, *Missions Will Not Impoverish the Country, Missionary Paper No. XI, American Board of Foreign Missions* (Boston: Crocker and Brewster, 1831), 3–4.
26 One clear example would be found in the writings of Elias Boudinot. Boudinot was a delegate to the Continental Congress from New Jersey and served as the body's president from 1782–1783. In 1815, Boudinot wrote a book (over 500 pages in length) laying out his beliefs on the second coming of Christ. See Elias Boudinot, *The Second Advent. Or, Coming of the Messiah in Glory, Shown to be a Scriptural Doctrine, and Taught by Divine Revelation from the Beginning of the World* (Trenton, NJ: Fenton & Hutchinson, 1815). Richard Lee Rogers describes Boudinot's efforts to convert Jews in America to Christianity as an example of his millennialist fervor. See Rogers, p. 45.
27 McDougall (1997), p. 18.
28 Ibid., p. 6.
29 Exploring these issues in depth is beyond the scope of this project. For a summary, see McDougall (1997), pp. 26–30.
30 Hutchison, pp. 5–6; 38–42.
31 Charles I. Foster, *An Errand of Mercy: The Evangelical United Front, 1790–1837* (Chapel Hill: University of North Carolina Press, 1960), 120–122.
32 Kimball and Beecher. Quote from p. 2.
33 Shenk, p. 3.
34 America's victory in the war did not lead to a fundamental break in the "special relationship" between the two countries, but it did re-enforce the theological claim that America had not taken

over the mantle of Christian faithfulness that the Church in Britain had squandered, reflecting the common belief (expressed in both theological and political frameworks) of American exceptionalism. For further discussion of the effects of the War of 1812 on American foreign missions and on the foreign policy of the country, see David Kling, "The New Divinity and the Origins of the ABCFM," in *North American Foreign Missions*, 1810–1914, William R. Shenk, ed. (Grand Rapids, MI: Eerdmans Publishing, 2004), 11–38. Also, see McDougall (1997), pp. 34–36.

35 Hutchison, quoting Griffin, p. 56.

36 Kling, p. 27.

37 For a fascinating history of the social reforms espoused by Evangelicals in general and Evangelicals in the American South in particular, see Leigh Heyrman, *Southern Cross: The Beginnings of the Bible Belt* (New York: Alfred Knopf, 1997).

38 James Monroe, *Seventh Annual Message to the United States Congress* (speech, Washington, DC, December 2, 1823), The American Presidency Project, www.presidency.ucsb.edu/ws/index.php?pid=29465, accessed January 26, 2018.

39 McDougall (1997), p. 83.

40 Expansionism did not spark only after the 1812 victory. Senior government leaders had set the stage for an aggressive expansionist streak from the founding of the new nation when Benjamin Franklin insisted for a Western boundary for the nation stretching all the way to the Mississippi River in the Treaty of Paris in 1781. President Thomas Jefferson expanded the nation's land holdings with the Louisiana Purchase in 1803, and President John Quincy Adams argued that "North America seems destined by Divine Providence to be peopled by one nation, speaking one language, professing one general system of religious and political principles, and accustomed to one general tenor of social usages and customs." (Quoted in McDougall (1997), p. 78) For an in-depth analysis of expansionism on American identity and its foreign policy, see McDougall (1997), chapter four.

41 Hutchison, p. 46.

42 John O'Sullivan, "The Great Nation of Futurity," in *The United States Democratic Review* 6, no. 23 (1845): 426–430. Italics added.

43 In 1836, the Mexican state of Coahuila was granted independence from Mexico after American settlers moved in to outnumber the Mexican residents by a factor of eight to one. This territory was not granted statehood as Texas until 1844. See McDougall (1997), pp. 90–93.

44 Matthew Niederhuber, "The Fight Over Innoculation During the 1721 Boston Smallpox Epidemic. Science in the News. Online: http://sitn.hms.harvard.edu/flash/special-edition-on-infectious-disease/2014/the-fight-over-inoculation-during-the-1721-boston-smallpox-epidemic/, accessed January 18, 2018).

45 Ann M. Becker, "Inoculation in Washington's Army: The Battle Against Smallpox," in *Science in Uniform, Uniforms in Science: Historical Studies of the American Military and Scientific Interactions*, eds. Margaret Vining and Barton Hacker (Washington: Smithsonian National Museum of American History, 2007), 20.

46 Richard Gabriel and Karen Metz, *A History of Military Medicine* (New York: Greenwood Press, 1992), 107.

47 For a discussion of the discovery of the Smallpox vaccine and its importance for public health, see Bess Furman, *A Profile of the United States Public Health Service 1798–1948* (Washington: U.S. Department of Health, Education, and Welfare, 1973). pp. 15–43. The term vaccination is derived from the Latin word vacca, or cow, in reference to the cowpox vaccine.

48 Furman, p. iii. The front matter of the book contains a photograph of the original 1798 act.

49 Furman, p. 12.

50 Ibid., p. 54.

51 John S. Chambers, *The Conquest of Cholera* (New York: Macmillan, 1938), 19.

52 Furman, pp. 52–53.

53 Samuel Jackson, "Report Embracing a View of the Principal Facts Connected with the Prevalence of Malignant Cholera in Philadelphia in 1832, Made to the Consulting Medical Board," in *The Cholera Gazette* I, no. 16 (1832): 252.

54 The story of that cholera outbreak and the responses of Snow and Whitehead can be found in the book The Ghost Map. See Steven Johnson, *The Ghost Map: The Story of London's Most Terrifying*

Epidemic – and How it Changed Sciences, Cities, and the Modern World (New York: Penguin, 2006). The American Epidemiological Society has adopted as its symbol a piece of London's wooden water pipe system that was replaced after the outbreak occurred and the Council of State and Territorial Epidemiologists awards its "Pumphandle Awards" to one person each year for "outstanding achievement in the field of applied epidemiology."

55 The account is referenced in Furman, p. 53.

56 For a discussion on the medical care provided by Methodist clergy in the 1700 and 1800s, see Karen Scheib, "John Wesley's 'Sensible Regimen' and 'Primitive Physick," in *Religion as a Social Determinant of Public Health*, ed. Ellen Idler (New York: Oxford University Press, 2014), 113–132.

57 Hutchison, p. 80.

58 Furman, pp. 82–85.

59 The definitive text that frames the work of the ACS as a supporter of abolition and traces its founding to Reverend Finley is P.J. Staudenraus, *The American Colonization Movement, 1816–1865* (New York: Columbia University Press, 1961). More recent historical interpretations have argued that the ACS both in its purpose and its impact was far more ambiguous. See Douglas R. Egerton, "'Its Origin is Not a Little Curious': A New Look at the American Colonization Society," in *The Journal of the Early Republic* 5, no. 4 (1985): 463–480. Egerton argues that the impetus for the founding of ACS came from Charles Mercer as the result of his fears that freed slaves and other members of poor and working classes were a pre-eminent threat to the newly industrializing society.

60 C.C. Goen, *Broken Churches, Broken Nation: Denominational Schisms and the Coming of the American Civil War* (Macon, GA: Mercer University Press, 1985).

References

Becker, Ann M. "Inoculation in Washington's Army: The Battle Against Smallpox." In *Science in Uniform, Uniforms in Science: Historical Studies of the American Military and Scientific Interactions*, eds. Margaret Vining and Barton Hacker, 15–32. Washington: Smithsonian National Museum of American History, 2007.

Boudinot, Elias. *The Second Advent. Or, Coming of the Messiah in Glory, Shown to be a Scriptural Doctrine, and Taught by Divine Revelation from the Beginning of the World.* Trenton, NJ: Fenton & Hutchinson, 1815.

Chambers, John S. *The Conquest of Cholera*. New York: Macmillan, 1938.

Crosby, Alfred. *Ecological Imperialism: The Biological Expansion of Europe, 900- 1900*. Cambridge, MA: Cambridge University Press, 1986.

Deichman Edwards, Wendy J. "Forging an Ideology for American Missions: Josiah Strong and Manifest Destiny." In *North American Foreign Missions, 1810–1914*, ed. William R. Shenk, 163–191. Grand Rapids, MI: Eerdmans Publishing, 2004.

Egerton, Douglas R. "'Its Origin is Not a Little Curious': A New Look at the American Colonization Society." *The Journal of the Early Republic* 5, no. 4 (1985): 463–480.

Eliot, John. *New England's First Fruits; In Respect, First of the Conversion of Some, Conviction of Divers, Preparation of Sundry of the Indians*. London: Henry Overton, 1643.

__________. *The Christian Commonwealth: Or, The Civil Policy Of The Rising Kingdom of Jesus Christ*. London: Liverwell Chapman, 1659.

Emmons, Nathanael. *A Sermon, Preached on the Annual Thanksgiving in Massachusetts. November 27, 1800*. Wrentham, MA: Nathaniel Heaton, 1801.

Foster, Charles I. *An Errand of Mercy: The Evangelical United Front, 1790–1837*. Chapel Hill: University of North Carolina Press, 1960.

Furman, Bess. *A Profile of the United States Public Health Service 1798–1948*. Washington: U.S. Department of Health, Education, and Welfare, 1973.

Gabriel, Richard and Karen Metz. *A History of Military Medicine*. New York: Greenwood Press, 1992.

Goes, C. C. *Broken Churches, Broken Nation: Denominational Schisms and the Coming of the American Civil War*. Macon, GA: Mercer University Press, 1985.

Heyrman, Leigh. *Southern Cross: The Beginnings of the Bible Belt*. New York: Alfred Knopf, 1997.

Hutchison, William R. *Errand to the World: American Protestant Thought and Foreign Missions*. Chicago: University of Chicago Press, 1987.

Jackson, Samuel. "Report Embracing a View of the Principal Facts Connected with the Prevalence of Malignant Cholera in Philadelphia in 1832, Made to the Consulting Medical Board." *The Cholera Gazette* I, no. 16 (1832): 244–252.

Johnson, Steven. *The Ghost Map: The Story of London's Most Terrifying Epidemic—and How It Changed Sciences, Cities, and the Modern World*. New York: Penguin, 2006.

Kimball, D. T. and Lyman Beecher. *Missions Will Not Impoverish the Country, Missionary Paper No. XI, American Board of Foreign Missions*. Boston: Crocker and Brewster, 1831.

Kling, David. "The New Divinity and the Origins of the ABCFM." In *North American Foreign Missions, 1810–1914*, ed. William R. Shenk, 11–38. Grand Rapids, MI: Eerdmans Publishing, 2004.

Mather, Cotton. *Magnalia Christi Americana or The Ecclesial History of New England, Vols. I and II*, ed. Kenneth B. Murdock. Cambridge, MA: Belknap Press of Harvard University Press, 1977.

McDougall, Walter A. *Promised Land, Crusader State: The American Encounter with the World Since 1776*. New York: Houghton Mifflin, 1997.

Monroe, James. "Seventh Annual Message to the United States Congress." Speech, Washington, DC, December 2, 1823. The American Presidency Project, www.presidency.ucsb.edu/ws/index.php?pid=29465. Accessed January 26, 2018.

Moore, Martin. *Memoirs of the Life and Character of Rev. John Eliot, Apostle of the N.A. Indians*. Boston: Flagg & Gould, 1822.

Niederhuber, Matthew. "The Fight Over Inoculation During the 1721 Boston Smallpox Epidemic." Science in the News. http://sitn.hms.harvard.edu/flash/special-edition-on-infectious-disease/2014/the-fight-over-inoculation-during-the-1721-boston-smallpox-epidemic/. Accessed January 18, 2018.

O'Sullivan, John. "The Great Nation of Futurity." *The United States Democratic Review* 6, no. 23 (1845): 426–430.

Rogers, Richard Lee. "A Bright and New Constellation: Millennial Narratives and the Origins of American Foreign Missions." In *North American Foreign Missions, 1810–1914*, ed. William R. Shenk, 39–60. Grand Rapids, MI: Eerdmans Publishing, 2004.

Rubin, Julius H. *Tears of Repentance: Christian Indian Identity and Community in Colonial Southern New England*. Lincoln, NE: University of Nebraska Press, 2013.

Salisbury, Neal. *Manitou and Providence: Indians, Europeans, and the Making of New England, 1500–1643*. New York: Oxford University Press, 1982.

Scheib, Karen. "John Wesley's 'Sensible Regimen' and 'Primitive Physick'." In *Religion as a Social Determinant of Public Health*, ed. Ellen Idler, 113–132. New York: Oxford University Press, 2014.

Shenk, Wilbert R. "Introduction." In *North American Foreign Missions, 1810–1914*, ed. William R. Shenk, 1–10. Grand Rapids, MI: Eerdmans Publishing, 2004.

Stannard, David E. *American Holocaust: The Conquest of the New World*. New York: Oxford University Press, 1992.

Staudenraus, P. J. *The American Colonization Movement, 1816–1865*. New York: Columbia University Press, 1961.

Walker, Williston. "Massachusetts and the Saybrook Platform." *Yale Historical Review* 1, no. 1 (1892): 69–86.

Winthrop, John. "A Model of Christian Charity." In *The Journals of John Winthrop*, eds. Richard S. Dunn and Laetitia Yeandle, 1–12. Cambridge, MA: The Belknap Press of Harvard University Press, 1996.

2 "Christianity is adequate to the work"

Religion and social reform in the progressive era

As the City Inspector for the City of New York from 1842–1843 and the Chief Physician of the City Hospital in New York from 1843–1870, John Griscom saw firsthand the social issues and health challenges facing New York's inhabitants in the middle of the nineteenth century. Cholera, yellow fever, and other infections were common and widespread; illiteracy was high; rapidly expanding factories had little to no regulation in their working conditions; and a burgeoning immigrant population in the city was being squeezed into tenement buildings where living conditions were poor and alcoholism and poverty were abundant. Griscom believed he had a duty to address these circumstances, and his efforts represent some of the first public health programs in the United States.

In response, he developed initiatives that addressed social and environmental conditions such as air quality, unregulated housing that left too many of the city's poorer citizens in sub-standard and unsafe conditions, and the periodic epidemics that befell the city.[1] In carrying out these initiatives, Griscom was one of the first to describe the distinction between medicine and public health:

> It is necessary to understand the distinction between *Public Health* and *Individual Health*. . . . The difference depends chiefly on the cause being *personal* or *general*. Thus an individual may be made sick by causes which affect no one else . . . and yet even these diseases, personal and peculiar as they seem to be, will sometimes be found dependent upon causes which affect large numbers at the same time. . . . In such cases, a well-directed inquiry into the condition in which people live, the position and arrangement of their working and lodging rooms, the character of their food, their habits of dress and cleanliness, the well or ill ventilated rooms they occupy by day and by night, would . . . fully account for the great and premature mortality of our citizens.[2]

Even as John Griscom was developing governmental initiatives aimed at improving the health of the New York's citizens, Robert Milham Hartley founded the New York Association for Improving the Condition of the Poor, one of the nation's first social service organizations, in 1842. While Griscom was addressing the poor health among the citizens of New York as a physician, Hartley attempted to address social factors. The purpose of Hartley's Association was to:

> advance the social, moral, and material interests of large masses of the community [to] provide for existing difficulties, avoid known evils, and secure beneficent results. It contemplated escaping the evils inseparable from isolated and independent exertions, through the united and concerted action of a general organization; hoping thus to diminish the chances of imposition, to ascertain the exact amount of charity each individual received, and to secure its judicious distribution. Moral means were to be employed, from the fact that no other would be adequate to produce the results, which the condition of the indigent required. It contemplated likewise preventive rather than remedial measures. It was primarily and directly to discountenance indiscriminate alms giving; to visit the poor at their homes, to give them counsel, to assist them when practicable in obtaining employment, to inspire them with self-respect and self-reliance, to inculcate habits of economy, industry, and temperance, and whenever absolutely necessary to provide such relief as should be suited to their wants.[3]

Two men were working independently in the same city (the nation's largest) for the first time to develop city-wide initiatives to improve health. Griscom, a medical doctor, was also a devout Quaker. Hartley, a successful businessman, was also a devout Presbyterian. Their efforts offer an early glimpse into the field of public health that was first starting to emerge in the United States. Their efforts also demonstrate that those same public health efforts were directly connected to the social and theological worldview of American Protestantism. From the beginning, the religion played a role both in supporting a moral framework for diagnosing the cause of the social ills and for offering a remedy. Griscom and Hartley believed that pauperism was the source of the ills facing their city. From the perspective of this nineteenth-century idea, the poverty so pervasive in New York was caused by an individual's moral weakness—the poor were responsible for their station because of their weak moral fiber. Christianity (specifically Protestantism) provided the only moral force sufficient to overcome pauperism. Hartley's own words reflect these two perspectives:

> Official data show, though imperfectly, how large a part of the pauperism of the City and State is occasioned by indolence, intemperance, and other vices; and were the returns full and accurate, and the effects closely followed up to their origin, it would doubtless appear that there is very little pauperism amongst us not directly or indirectly traceable to these and kindred sources. To remove the evil we must remove the causes; and these being chiefly moral—whatever subsidiary appliances may be used—they admit only moral remedies. Make the individuals composing the great mass of paupers industrious, sober, virtuous, and the work of social regeneration will be effected; while any attempted

> social reform which excludes such a change of character, would be to lop off the branches of the Upas, and leave the poisonous root to shoot out with more baneful luxuriance.[4]

As a chemist, Griscom's father helped establish the medical school at Rutgers University; he also helped found the American Bible Society in 1816 and the Society for the Prevention of Pauperism in 1817.[5] In his father's biography, John Griscom summarized the Society's position of moral weakness as the root cause of pauperism:

> The causes [of pauperism] were stated to be,
>
> 1st, *Ignorance.*
> 2d, *Idleness.*
> 3d, *Intemperance in drinking,*—"emphatically the *cause of causes;* the box of Pandora is realized in each keg of ardent spirit that stands upon the counters of the 1,600 licensed grocers of this city."
> 4th, *Want of Economy.*
> 5th, *Imprudent and hasty marriages.*
> 6th, *Lotteries.*
> 7th, *Pawnbrokers.*
> 8th, *Houses of ill-fame.*
> 9th, *The numerous charitable institutions of the city.*
> 10th, *War,* "during its prevalence one of the most abundant sources of poverty and vice."[6]

The idea that those who were poor bore the primary responsibility for their condition would remain. Seventy-five years after the founding of the Society for the Prevention of Pauperism, John Shaw Billings, one of the key leaders in establishing the field of public health in the United States and champion of the U.S. Public Health Service, echoed the perspectives of the society while also making explicit connections between pauperism and race:

> Pauperism consists of a distinct class of people who are structurally and almost necessarily idle, ignorant, intemperate, and more or less vicious, who are failures, or the descendants of failures, and who for the most part belong to certain races.[7]

Moral weakness was the cause (and "a distinct class of people" were most susceptible to that weakness). The moral strength and truth of Christianity provided the answer:

> If there is one kind of effort more to be deprecated than another, it is that which attempts the reform of deep-seated social evils, without the agency

> of the only power adequate to their eradication—the moral spirit of Christianity . . . Whatever is done for the relief of the great mass of the degraded poor, without a reform of character, renders them not only more exacting and dependent, but actually multiplies in themselves and in their offspring the evils designed to be removed . . . The work is vast and difficult, and will require time for its accomplishment. It is a work in which all mere human devices have signally failed, and ever will fail. But it will yield to the divine method. The supernatural efficiency of Christianity is adequate to the work . . . The social problem, in short, finds a practical solution in the principles of Christianity, as set forth in the teachings, and illustrated by the example of Christ and his Apostles.[8]

But how would the good news of Christian morality be spread to this "distinct class of people?" Hartley found the answer to that question: Christian tracts. As an officer in the New York chapter of the American Tract Society, Hartley used the activities of the New York Association for the Improving the Condition of the Poor to spread the (health) gospel contained in the tracts:

> The Association began the issuing of tracts, designed to inform the more unfortunate in the community what was expected of them, though they were poor; how to conduct themselves in their poverty; what to adopt, what to avoid; how to buy, cook, economize; in a word, how to live—live happily, live successfully . . . We would merely mention some of the more prominent of these topics, that received consideration and were given to the public. Street Begging and Vagrancy; The Proper Subjects of Charity; Domestic Economy; Food and Drink, with the best Modes of Preparation; Plans for the Better Distribution of Medical Attendance and Medicines for the Indigent Sick, but the Public Dispensaries of the City; Sanitary Law; Truancy; Sewerage; Employment; Apprentices; Dwellings; Widows; Orphans; Tenements; Crowded Dwellings; Public Health; Reformatories, and numerous others; all bearing upon the objects of the Association.[9]

Tract societies bridged the moral message of a nineteenth-century Protestant Christianity and practical health and social support information written expressly to address the living situations of the poor. More than 20 years before medical organizations in the United States developed coordinated public health responses, Thomas Hartley established "the most coherent and far-seeing public health program of any benevolent group while medical societies still concerned themselves marginally with such matters."[10] This was a thoroughly American response to a public health issue, but it had roots in foreign missions, and the approach spread to influence foreign mission efforts in subsequent years.

England had been the home of the tract movement beginning in the late eighteenth century. Initially, these tracts offered a standard fictional account of sinners encountering Jesus and finding salvation through confession of faith in him. However, by the 1810s, the subjects of British tracts had begun to address societal concerns such as pauperism, and the tract movement had spread around the world. The missionary effort of British Protestants to spread the gospel was emulated by other Christian bodies (and expanded, in the case of American Protestants) all across the globe. In the United States, missionary activity offered a means for tract distribution and missionary zeal powered the movement.[11]

By 1832, the American Tract Society was publishing close to 700 titles out of its Boston offices. The tract society focused its efforts in both domestic and international circles. Domestically, it offered materials in six different languages with a total circulation of over 15,000,000 copies,[12] a truly astounding number at a time when the nation's entire population was approximately 13,000,000.[13] Internationally, the tracts were key instruments in the work of the ABCFM.[14] By 1838, the Society published 418 different publications for use in foreign missions, ranging from single tracts to large, bound volumes for distribution abroad and to Native American communities in the United States. Those titles were published in 30 different languages: French, Spanish, German, Italian, Portuguese, Welsh, Cherokee, Choctaw, Mohawk, Seneca, Chippeway, Delaware Indian, Creole, Negro German, Hawaiian, Spanish, French, Armenian, Greek, Arabic, Afrikaans, Tamul, Mahratta, Orissa, Persian, Burmese, Siamese, Asamese, Chinese, and Japanese. The society described tract distribution in countries: China, Singapore, Burmah, Siam [present-day Thailand], Orissa [in present-day India], Tamul [in present-day India], Mahrattas [in present-day India], Northern India, Sandwich Islands [present-day Hawaii], Syria, Nestorians [part of present-day Turkey], Greece, Russia, Constantinople [part of present-day Turkey], France, South Africa, and the West Indies.[15]

The efforts of John Griscom and Robert Hartley to address the health conditions of the poorer residents of New York City represent an early example of the intersection of religion and public health in America. Those efforts were supported by a missionary zeal and by racist and classist beliefs about people who were not of Anglo-Saxon heritage. Religion was not the sole driver of such attitudes; rather, those attitudes were pervasive among religious leaders, health practitioners such as John Shaw Billings, and most people of higher educational and socio-economic status. The pervasiveness of such attitudes does not make them any less repugnant. Such attitudes impacted foreign missions, including medical missions, during this period, as we shall see. Finally, the zeal with which missionary tracts were distributed offers a concrete example of the social force of the Protestant missionary movement in the United States in the nineteenth century. This example of the public health missionary work of Griscom and Hartley, then, provides a context for examining foreign missions in the era.

In 1869, British foreign missionaries outnumbered their American counterparts by a ratio of greater than two to one. Over the next 30 years, that ratio reversed, and by the start of the twentieth century, the number of American foreign missionaries was more than double that of the British, and American Protestants were providing more funds to the foreign mission effort than were the British.[16] In 1870, American Protestants supported fewer than 20 medical or educational facilities as part of their foreign missions activities, but by 1902, there were 379 hospitals and 782 dispensaries run by American and European missionaries worldwide, along with 94 colleges and universities and 20,4558 schools.[17] Such growth would not have occurred without a concurrent growth in medical knowledge and technical capacities,[18] but it was missionary and not medical zeal that fueled efforts to employ these new technologies globally. This period of explosive growth occurred without any governmental funding for health and development initiatives; in fact, the present-day fields of global health and social development were started by Christian missionaries. Missionary health facilities would predate any facilities by the colonial governments that occupied most of the nations of Africa by decades, and missionaries were operating health facilities at least 30 years before any colonial health administrators were in place.[19]

This period of growth begs the question: why did medical missions become such a priority among broader missions' endeavors in the last half of the nineteenth century? In fact, this was simply a new context for a question that had been part of foreign mission endeavors for well over a century: did missions exist only to tell the story of the Christian gospel to those who had not heard it, or did it also have a purpose of caring for those in need?

Missions in the progressive era

Expanding the purpose of missions

Hartley and Griscom endeavored to address their country's pressing public health needs by relying on a Christian moral vision they hoped to establish in American society. This theological vision understood salvation not as the rescue of an individual's soul from sin and hellfire, but as the dawn of God's kingdom on earth ushered in through an American society that had overcome its various social ills by turning toward the truths of Christianity. This theology had a profound impact on American Protestantism in the nineteenth and early twentieth centuries, forming the base for a broad-based movement of social reform known as the Social Gospel.

Walter Rauschenbusch, an American Baptist theologian, was a primary spokesperson for the movement. Rauschenbusch made a theological case for the social gospel, arguing that it represented the continuation of the gospel narratives of Jesus's work of healing and care for the poor. According to this movement, the mark of faith was not an individualized, sentimental testimony to God's salvation from personal sinful transgression as much as a manifestation of God's thirst for justice in which those without have plenty and the society is transformed by God's redeeming love. Anticipating both the possibilities and the challenges facing the movement, Rauschenbusch wondered how those in the future would see the modern society of the late nineteenth century. Would they:

> describe the nineteenth and twentieth centuries as the golden age when outwardly life flourished as never before, but when that decay, which resulted in the gradual collapse of the twenty-first and twenty-second centuries, was already far advanced.
>
> Or will the twentieth century mark for the future historian the real adolescence of humanity, the great emancipation from barbarism and from the paralysis of injustice, and the beginning of a progress in the intellectual, social, and moral life of mankind to which all past history has no parallel?
>
> It will depend almost wholly on the moral forces which the Christian nations can bring to the fighting line against wrong, and the fighting energy of those moral forces will again depend on the degree to which they are inspired by religious faith and enthusiasm.[20]

Protestants in the nineteenth century clearly believed that missions had that dual purpose and was not solely focused on proselytization. This commitment, of course, had a series of implications: were medicine and education instruments to be used in support of the primary goal of conversion, or were they legitimate goals on their own to be offered without regard to the religious belief of those who received these services? How did medical and educational missionaries relate to the cultures of the people to whom they provided their services?

These questions generated sharp debates (in fact, they still do). Initially, medicine and education were seen instrumentally—offering them was a means to achieving a primary purpose of conversion to the Christian faith.[21] One missionary manual dictated the construction of the chapel before the construction of the hospital on the grounds of the new medical missions compounds,[22] while another mandated attendance at Christian worship services as a prerequisite to receiving medical care.[23] When medicine and education were aligned with introduction of the Christian religion to those who had not heard of it, missionary narratives spoke eloquently of the benefit of missions to human souls and human bodies:

> The evangelization of the world depends on the indigenous people of each nation, and what better missionary could be found than the leper cured of his disease, going back to his people telling them out of the fullness of his heart, the twofold gospel of spiritual and physical healing.[24]

Such alignment, however, was not always evident.

Some Protestants saw little need for medical or educational mission, believing that "faith and prayer was sufficient to insure native health."[25] Others were convinced that offering medical care as a goal in and of itself was a legitimate expression of their faith. Albert Schweitzer's medical missionary work is often named as an example of this perspective by those who argue that "he personified a new approach to Africa's suffering and poverty."[26] Although Scweitzer did not work until the early twentieth century, his writing does reflect such a perspective and represents an articulation of a perspective that predates him.

If the debate about medical missions in the 1840s focused on the question of whether its purpose was saving bodies or saving souls[27] over the next 40 years, mainline Protestants by and large came to see the provision of medical care and the establishment of schools as a worthy activity of their missionary endeavors if carried out in the service of evangelism. Medical missions became the "heavy artillery" of evangelism with the new technical knowledge mobilized for the purpose of conversion.[28] In 1905, the influential Protestant leader John Mott summarized this position:

> The value of medical, educational, literary, and all other forms of missionary activity, is measured by the extent to which they prepare the way for the Gospel message, promote its acceptance, manifest its spirit and benefits, multiply points of contact with human souls and increase the number and efficacy of those who preach Christ.[29]

For Mott, medical work was "one of the powerful, effective, and directly evangelistic agencies which the Church possesses."[30]

For the first 200 years of the British colonies and the first decades of the American nation, foreign missions had been carried in an explicitly evangelistic frame—it preached the gospel to "the heathen" to give them the opportunity to profess a saving knowledge of Jesus Christ so that they might achieve salvation. As technology opened up possibilities for rapid advancements in the practice of clinical medicine, the urgency of conversion was replaced with a desire to offer compassionate care to "the poor." Medical care became a key part of missions endeavors years before governmental or secular public health or clinical initiatives in global health or development. But such efforts were tied to America's expansionist ambitions and reflected in blatantly racist attitudes expressed by many Protestant religious leaders without the slightest hint of self-consciousness.

A racialized version of social reform

Foreign missions, including medical missions, was inextricably linked to an ever-stronger perception that America's manifest destiny was to save the world by remaking it in the nation's own image and to an idea that the "American" image was seen in the white, Anglo-Saxon, Protestant male.

When it was published in 1859, *The Origin of Species* upended scientific, religious, and social assumptions. Charles Darwin's book offered a thesis on the biological processes by which the astounding variety of animal life came to be. His theory of evolution countered the default assumptions of European culture regarding cosmology, divine creation, and the unique place of human beings in that creation. For the first 15 years after its publication, most Protestant theologians and pastors in the United States were united in their opposition, denouncing the book's scientific claims on the basis of their theological implications. The Congregationalist theologian Horace Bushnell wrote in 1868 that proof of the validity of Darwin's claims would lead Christians to the conclusion that "we may well enough agree to live without religion."[31] In fact, while Bushnell may have rejected Darwinism because it dethroned God as Creator with self-perpetuating biological processes, in time, his theological frameworks on race would be combined with a certain interpretation of Darwin's theories to articulate a racist vision of American Protestantism that many Social Gospel leaders embraced. Bushnell wrote that:

> Good principles and habits, intellectual culture, domestic virtues, industry, order, law, faith—all these go immediately to enhance the rate and capacity of population. They make a race powerful, not in the mere military sense, but in one that, by century-long reaches of populating force, lives down silently every mere martial competitor. Any people that is physiologically advanced in culture, though it be only in a degree, beyond another which is mingled with it on strictly equal terms, is sure to live down and live out its inferior. Nothing can save the inferior race but a ready and pliant assimilation. Christian salvation will become an inbred life and populating force, mighty enough to overlive, and finally to completely people the world. Inferior races will be over-populated and taken possession of by a truly sanctified stock.[32]

It is hardly surprising that this kind of theology would be joined with Darwinian biological theory to articulate a racist social vision grounded in biological language. Less than a decade after Bushnell wrote, as scientific assessments of Darwin's work supported his claims of the biological mechanisms at work, a growing number of theologians came to believe "it was necessary to accept the theory and to accommodate Christian theology to its dictates."[33] Many of those who came to accept Darwin avoided the theological implication of his biological claims but embraced his theory as a scientific framework that justified common racist preconceptions. For example, the Protestant minister Josiah Strong, a leading champion of the Social Gospel,[34] came to embrace Darwin's theory precisely because it provided a scientific framework onto which he could place such sociological and theological assumptions in his book *Our Country*:

> It is not unlikely that before the close of the next century, this [white] race will outnumber all the other civilized races of the world. Does it not look as if God

> were not only preparing in our Anglo-Saxon civilization the die with which to stamp the peoples of the earth, but as if he were also massing behind that die the mighty power with which to press it?
>
> The time is coming when the pressure of population on the means of subsistence will be felt here as it is now felt in Europe and Asia. Then will the world enter upon a new stage of its history—*the final competition of races, for which the Anglo-Saxon is being schooled*. Long before the thousand millions are here, the mighty *centrifugal* tendency, inherent in this stock and strengthened in the United States, will assert itself. Then this race of unequaled energy, with all the majesty of numbers and the might of wealth behind it—the representative, let us hope, of the largest liberty, the purest Christianity, the highest civilization—having developed peculiarly aggressive traits calculated to impress its institutions upon mankind, will spread itself over the earth. If I read not amiss, this powerful race will move down upon Mexico, down upon Central and South America, out upon the islands of the sea, over upon Africa and beyond. And can any one doubt that the result of this competition of races will be the "survival of the fittest"?[35]

Charles Darwin was invoked explicitly by Josiah Strong to bolster his claims:

> Mr. Darwin is not only disposed to see, in the natural vigor of our people, an illustration of his favorite theory of natural selection, but even intimates that the world's history thus far has been preparatory for our future, and tributary to it. He says: "There is apparently much truth in the belief that the wonderful progress of the United States, as well as the character of the people, are the results of natural selection; for the more energetic, restless, and courageous men from all parts of Europe have emigrated during the last ten or twelve generations to that great country and have there succeeded best."[36]

The kinds of racist views put forth by Strong were supported by Darwin's own colleagues. John Fiske, a strong proponent of Darwin's theories, argued that the United States possessed the precise combination of democracy, religion, and industry needed to peaceably civilize the world by introducing the stronger racial stock of the Anglo-Saxons and the superior culture of the United States and Europe. Darwin was a great admirer of Fiske. The two of them corresponded at length between 1871 and 1880 with 18 letters between them, and, upon Darwin's death, Fiske authored his ten-page obituary in *The Atlantic*.[37]

Our Country was a bestseller, with over 175,000 copies sold in its initial print run and the book was subsequently translated into Dutch and German. A revised version was published in 1891, again reaching bestseller status.[38] The book was actually a revision of an earlier series of works under the same title published by the American Home Missionary Society in 1858 and 1842—the first version being a much smaller tract that had laid out the Christian case for addressing the social needs of the poor. In the case of Robert Hartley, the alignment of social gospel zeal and concern for urban poverty had resulted in a public health response to improve living conditions. To the extent that such missionary tract efforts were grounded in notions of pauperism, they eventually gave rise to a "potpourri of evangelical Protestantism, vigorous nationalism, Social Darwinism, intense racialism, and American expansionism,"[39] reflected in Strong's writing.

Our Country not only espoused racist views, it reflected American nationalist tendencies by arguing for America's unique role to stand as a model to the world. Strong quotes a story that John Adams, the second President of the United States, told in his memoirs:

> John Adams records that nothing was "more ancient in his memory than the observation that arts, sciences and empire had traveled westward; and in conversation it was always added that their next leap would be over the Atlantic into America." He recalled a couplet that had been "inscribed, or rather drilled, into a rock on the shore of Monument Bay in our old colony of Plymouth: The Eastern nations sink, their glory ends, and empire rises where the sun descends."[40]

Expansionism, exceptionalism, racism, and theology combined in a way of thinking that influenced both American foreign policy in the political sphere and foreign missions in the religious sphere.

American colonialism and medical missions in the progressive era

The mechanisms of European colonization were at full force in the latter part of the nineteenth century. Colonization in Africa demonstrates the European nations' appetite for colonial expansion even though it was not the only continent on which such appetite fed. In 1870, European colonies comprised about 10% of Africa; by 1900, almost 90% of the continent's landmass was ruled by the European powers who had divided the continent among themselves at the Berlin Conference of 1884.[41] The provision of medical care—almost all of it carried out by missionaries—was part of the machinery of Empire, even as some missionaries raised pointed critiques, as we shall later see. Colonial medicine consisted of both mission and mandate. It had two missions—to spread Christianity through medical care and champion scientific rationality—and two mandates—to further colonial rule in the "uncivilized" lands and help consolidate that rule in the places where it had been established.[42] Government and church worked in support of colonization with missionaries building churches, schools, and medical facilities to serve the people who had their land taken from them by governmental and business forces. Appeals to churchgoers recruited them to the cause of keeping tropical colonies from becoming the "white man's grave" in order that the lands might be civilized by instituting European businesses and consolidating colonial rule.[43]

Similar processes had been unfolding in the United States, providing a justification for the westward push to the Pacific Coast as the nation claimed as its own the land that Native Americans had previously held for millennia. This claiming of others' lands by force had been part of the nation's history since the first Europeans came to the New World in the seventeenth century, and such violence was also accompanied by Christian missions that brought along schools, hospitals, and the structures of Western civilization. Nonetheless, Americans saw their own land grabs in a different light from Europe's colonization of lands in Africa and Asia. After all, Americans claimed that the lands being annexed into the country were on the same continent, God had clearly ordained those lands to be part of the nation, and America was not interested in conquering foreign lands. While it was true that the nation had established and maintained strategic bases in Alaska, Samoa, and Hawaii, those efforts had been in response to European aggression in the hemisphere and reflected the nation's commitment to following the Monroe Doctrine outlined in 1823. Apologists for a vision of America not influenced by empire argued that the United States maintained military bases in those nations but it did not set out to overthrow the existing governments and establish a colonial administration of its own. However, as the nation prepared for the start of the twentieth century, it would face the question of foreign intervention on lands off the North American continent.[44]

The era of American empire

In 1895, when some residents of the Spanish colony in Cuba rebelled, America's leaders were unsure how to respond. In general, the nation sympathized with the rebellion and expressed outrage at the response of the Spanish government when it removed villagers to camps. They also feared the health consequences of the Spanish attempts to quash the rebellion.

By 1897, when William McKinley entered office as the new American President, over 100,000 Cubans had died from disease and famine. Americans feared outbreaks of diseases from Cuba on American shores, since "Cuba had long been viewed as a hotbed of yellow fever and a source of the recurrent yellow fever epidemics that ravaged the American South" and "the invasion of Cuba was intended to put an end to this hemispheric threat of invasion."[45] As early as 1879, the U.S. National Board of Health had raised concerns about endemic disease in Cuba and the threat it represented for the United States. The Board's 1879 report described

> unpaved, garbage-ridden streets; poor, overcrowded housing that lacked ventilation; and the absence of proper sanitation. Most households relied on

> privies to dispose of human waste, which contaminated the soil and the city's water supply. Referring to the pervasive use of privies, the report noted: "The effluvia therefrom pervades the houses, and the fluid contents saturate the soil and the soft porous coral rocks on which the city is built. Hence, all well water is ruined, and every ditch dug in the streets exhales an offensive odor. Thus Havana may be said to be built over a privy."[46]

Many religious leaders, including some of the nation's most prominent Protestant pastors and advocates for the Social Gospel, rallied in support of Cuban independence, even if it meant armed conflict with Spain. American historian Walter McDougall notes:

> Protestant journals made noises like this: "And if it be the will of Almighty God that by war the last trace of this inhumanity of man to man shall be swept away from this Western hemisphere, let it come!" And this: "Should we now go to war our cause will be just. Every Methodist preacher will be a recruiting officer." . . . And *The Churchman* warned: "Woe to any nation . . . called to guide a weaker people's future which hesitates for fear its own interests will be entangled and its own future imperiled by the discharge of an unmistakeable *[sic]* duty."[47]

What was McKinley to do? To actively intervene would risk war with Spain and represent America's refusal to honor its own position articulated in the Monroe Doctrine, but the deaths and suffering on the island struck America's conscience, and the destruction of American property on the island struck America's wallet. Finally, McKinley felt compelled to intervene, especially when he learned that Spain was seeking financial support for its occupation from other European governments.[48] On April 11, 1898, McKinley requested authorization from Congress to use force in the protection of U.S. interests on the island and end the war "in the cause of humanity."[49]

The Congress refused McKinley's request for war but instead issued a joint resolution recognizing Cuban independence and authorizing the President to use force to ensure that this independence was respected by other nations. Members of Congress could thereby frame their decision not as aggression but as furthering the spirit of democracy and a compassionate response to a neighbor in need, a perspective articulated by Senator John Spooner when he said,

> we intervene not for conquest, not for aggrandizement, not because of the Monroe Doctrine; we intervene for humanity's sake . . . to aid a people who have suffered every form of tyranny and who have made a desperate struggle to be free.[50]

The United States entered into war against Spain in 1898, and the conflict spread beyond Cuba to other Spanish colonial territories.

Fighting was short-lived, with a ceasefire in August of 1898, four months after the conflict began, and America, for the first time in its history, had carried out armed conflict on foreign soil in a context in which its own sovereignty was not at stake. How to justify this decision? And what to do with the lands of Cuba, Guam, Puerto Rico, and the Philippines that were now independent of Spain and under American control? What was America to make of its new role as a colonial, occupying power? It would take a few years and hundreds of thousands of deaths in the Philippines to answer this question.

The United States determined that the people of the Philippines were unprepared for self-rule, and, since the war had been predicated on a response to the cruelty of Spanish colonialism, the United States was unsure what to do next. Sentiment in America was strong for annexation of the nation.[51] Following a "prayerful night," President McKinley decided that

> there was nothing for us to do but take them all, and to educate the Filipinos, and uplift and civilize and Christianize them, and by God's grace do the very best we could by them, as our fellow-men for whom Christ also died.

This statement of self-proclaimed beneficence accompanied coercion by McKinley as well. This process of Christianization/Americanization of the Philippines required that the Filipinos "come to see our benevolent purpose and recognize that before we can give their people good government our sovereignty must be complete and unquestioned."[52]

Washington Gladden, a national leader in the Social Gospel movement, called the liberation of Cuba and the colonization of the Philippines "an act of friendship."[53] It seems that someone forgot to tell this to the Filipinos themselves. The treaty ending the war transferred governmental control of the colony from the Spanish to the American government in 1899. Two days before the treaty signing, Filipino rebels shot at American soldiers, who returned fire. A day later, there were 3,000 Philippine and 59 Americans casualties; six months after the end of the Spanish-American War, the Philippine-American War had begun. John Fiske, the evolutionary philosopher favored by many proponents of the Social Gospel, argued that "war would continue until the barbarous races were all subdued, since for them, war was both a necessity and a favorite occupation."[54] The war would continue until 1902, when President Theodore Roosevelt[55] declared an end to conflict and confirmed that U.S. rule over the nation had come to an end. The day was July 4; America and the Philippines would share the same national day commemorating their independence. The war would eventually result in the deaths of over 200,000 Filipinos and 5,000 Americans, costing over $400,000,000 (over $30 billion when adjusted for inflation to 2008 monetary levels).[56]

The precedent set by the nation's armed conflict against Spain became a new policy—the Roosevelt corollary to the Monroe Doctrine. Speaking to both houses of Congress in the 1904 State of the Union address, President Roosevelt set forth a new position: the nation had both a right and a duty to pre-emptively intervene in the affairs of another nation if that nation's actions might present a threat to America's self-interests:

> It is not true that the United States feels any land hunger or entertains any projects as regards the other nations of the Western Hemisphere save such as are for their welfare. All that this country desires is to see the neighboring countries stable, orderly, and prosperous. If a nation shows that it knows how to act with reasonable efficiency and decency in social and political matters, if it keeps order and pays its obligations, it need fear no interference from the United States. Chronic wrongdoing, or an impotence which results in a general loosening of the ties of civilized society, may in America, as elsewhere, ultimately require interventions by some civilized nation, and in the Western Hemisphere the adherence of the United States to the Monroe Doctrine may force the United States, however reluctantly, in flagrant cases of such wrongdoing or impotence, to the exercise of an *international police power* . . . We would interfere with them only as a last resort, and then only if it became evident that their unwillingness to do justice at home and abroad had violated the rights of the United States or had invited foreign aggression to the detriment of the entire body of American nations.[57]

Roosevelt explicitly invoked the Monroe Doctrine on multiple occasions in articulating his foreign policy position, never acknowledging the irony of predicating a justification for America's right to intervene militarily even in the absence of an overt act of aggression on a doctrine that warns other nations not to intervene in nations, lands, or territories of the Western Hemisphere. The irony seems to have been lost on many; in 1906, he was awarded the Nobel Peace Prize.

Senior leaders of the Social Gospel, such as Washington Gladden, Walter Rauschenbusch, and Josiah Strong, all decried America's brief foray into imperialism and its colonial rule of the Philippines. At the same time, they strongly supported the nation's military intervention there and the decision to take up arms against Spain. These Social Gospelers were key contributors to America's distinctive foreign policy at the time: temporary occupation and tutelage.[58] After the Philippines gained independence, American government personnel remained behind and American private investment was sent to build ports, roads, schools, hospitals, and railroads. With the new government in leadership, land reform and economic innovations were instituted: "It was imperialism, but a self-consciously progressive imperialism born of Americans' sense of secular and religious mission."[59] The colonization aspiration of the United States would not be in any way as comprehensive or long-standing as its European peers, but for Protestants in the nation, mission and mandate went hand in hand in ways that echoed Europe's mission efforts. For

American Protestant Christians, the mission was the Christianization of the social order in the mold of the Social Gospel,[60] and the mandate was the Americanization of the world's nations in order to fulfill America's godly destiny.

The connections between that mission and mandate led to a blurring of the liens between America's secular narrative and its (Protestant Christian) narrative. In large part:

> [Imperialism was driven by] the same do-gooder impulse that inspired the reforms of the Progressive Era within the United States. Colonial administrators, economists, teachers, doctors, missionaries, investors, and the Army Corps of Engineers descended on Cuba, the Philippines, Guam, and Panama to whip Yellow Fever, build the Panama Canal (which Roosevelt dubbed a gift to humanity), develop the economies, and free the people from their Spanish Catholic legacy.
>
> The belief that American power, guided by a secular and religious spirit of service, could remake foreign societies came as easily to the Progressives as trust-busting, prohibition of child labor, and regulation of interstate commerce, meatpacking, and drugs. Leading imperialists . . . were all Progressive; leading Progressives . . . were all imperialists.[61]

As America entered into the twentieth century, the nation seemed to possess a strong, unified optimism and confidence in the moral clarity of its religious, social, and political positions in both domestic and foreign affairs to transfer the empire of the world. Such optimism and confidence would not last and a unified vision would come undone in the first decades of the next century. Even as broad support for America's "progressive imperialism" was visible, discontent and different opinions were starting to arise. Writing in 1896, Walter Rauschenbusch encouraged the nation to re-double its efforts to fulfill its destiny in the Christianization of the social order and put aside differences between the religious and the secular as well as divides among Christian themselves:

> We believe in the spiritual life, in the fact of sin and corruption, in the need and possibility of salvation, in holiness and eternal life. We have no desire to see evangelical Christianity bled to death; to see the church of Christ turned into a reform club; to see the hidden life of the believer toned down to a mild and sapless altruism; and to have Christian theology changed into a modern gnosticism, into a system of evolutionary philosophy, with a place for Christ as one of the evolutionary forces. On the contrary, we find fault with modern Christianity because it is not Christian enough. We desire a completer surrender to the Spirit of God, a fuller life of trust, and a more ardent zeal for all missionary work, and for the universal reign of King Jesus. But, on the other hand, we also believe in the social movement of the nineteenth century. We

> refuse to regard it as a red-hot lava eruption from the crater of hell. We hold that it is a river flowing from the throne of God, sent by the Ruler of history for the purification of the nations. We see God's hand in it; we see Christ's blood in it; we see the creative energies of the Spirit in it, bringing out of its chaos the beauties of a new world.
>
> We have this two-sided faith. But our faith is not yet supported on all sides by knowledge. The two chemical elements have not yet completed their union in us. We must overhaul all the departments of our thought and work out that social Christianity which will be immeasurably more powerful and more valuable to the world than either an unsocial Christianity or an unchristian socialism.[62]

Rauschenbusch was trying to find ties that bound the culture and the church together even as the centrifugal forces of modernism were straining a common, universal commitment. The United States entered into the twentieth century as a global power and with a vision of its global role as compassionate champion of the poor, uneducated, and sick—a vision common among the nation's citizens even if others such as the Filipino citizens who had endured such violence during armed conflict with America did not share it. Commitment to that vision in the popular imagination of the country was possible only by overlooking key aspects of the nation's political power. For a while, those aspects would be covered over but in time, there could be no full and lasting resolution between such a vision and the nation's politics. A half century after Rauschenbusch exhorted the nation to find common cause, the United States would be negotiating its position in the aftermath of two global wars. These wars, the events leading up to them, and the decisions made after they ended would leave an indelible mark on American Protestantism and on the fields of public health and international development.

Notes

1 John Griscom, *The Sanitary Condition of the Laboring Poor of New York* (New York: Harper & Brothers, 1845).

2 Ibid., pp. 3–4. Italics in original text.

3 Isaac Smithson Hartley, *Memorial of Robert Milham Hartley* (New York: Arno Press, 1976 (1882)), 186–187.

4 Ibid., pp. 307–308. is making reference to the Upas Tree in Java. The tree's sap was believed to be poisonous according to a legend widely cited in the nineteenth century.

5 Rossiter Johnson and John Howard Brown, The Twentieth Century Biographical Dictionary of Notable Americans: Brief Biographies of Authors, Administrators, Clergymen, Commanders, Editors, Engineers, Jurists, Merchants, Officials, Philanthropists, Scientists, Statesmen, and Others Who Are Making American History, Volume IV: Ericsson-Gwin (Boston: The Biographical Society, 1904).

6 John Griscom, *Memoir of John Griscom, LL.D., Late Professor of Chemistry and Natural Philosophy* (New York: Robert Carter and Brothers, 1859), 159.

7 John Shaw Billings, *Public Health and Municipal Government: An Address Delivered Before the American Academy of Political and Social Science at the Art Club, Philadelphia, Jan. 14, 1891* (Philadelphia:

American Academy of Political and Social Science, 1891), 6. For a comprehensive history of Billings's role in the creation of the modern public health movement in the United States, see Bess Furman, *A Profile of the United States Public Health Service 1798–1948* (Washington: U.S. Department of Health, Education, and Welfare, 1973).

8 Hartley, pp. 307–310.

9 Hartley, pp. 197–200.

10 Charles E. Rosenberg and Carroll S. Rosenberg, "Pietism and the Origins of the American Public Health Movement: A Note on John H. Griscom and Robert M. Hartley in" *Journal of the History of Medicine and Allied Sciences* 23, no. 1 (January 1968): 31.

11 Samuel G. Green, *The Story of the Religious Tract Society for One Hundred Years* (London: The Religious Tract Society, 1899), 56–60.

12 See *Nineteenth Annual Report of the American Tract Society* (Boston: Perkins & Marvin, 1833).

13 The population of the United States according to the 1830 census was 12,858,670. See Abstract of the Returns of the Fifth Census, Showing the Number of Free People, the Number of Slaves, the Federal or Representative Numbers, and the Aggregate of Each County of Each State of The United States. Washington, DC: Dugg Green, 1832. Online: http://www2.census.gov/library/publications/decennial/1830/1830b.pdf, accessed January 22, 2018).

14 The ABCFM continued supporting mission work as an ecumenical body of various Protestant denominations for a number of years, but after the Civil War the denominations also began to sponsor their own missionaries. The scope of the foreign mission endeavor grew, but that work was no longer coordinated solely through the ABCFM. In time, individual denominational bodies grew larger, and, eventually, the ABCFM became the mission body of the Congregationalists. In 1961, the ABCFM merged with the Board of International Missions to form the United Church Board for World Ministries; this body was renamed the Wider Church Ministries of the United Church of Christ, a liberal Christian denomination that counts the Congregationalists as one of its founding bodies. For discussion on the splintering of the ABCFM in the 1960s, see William R. Hutchison, *Errand to the World: American Protestant Thought and Foreign Missions* (Chicago: University of Chicago Press, 1987), 95.

15 See *Twenty-Fourth Annual Report of the American Tract Society* (Boston: Perkins & Marvin, 1838).

16 Hutchison, p. 93.

17 Hutchison, p. 100

18 Charles M. Good, "Pioneer Medical Missions in Colonial Africa," in *Social Science and Medicine* 32, no. 1 (1991): 1–2.

19 Ibid., p. 1.

20 Walter Rauschenbusch, *Christianity and the Social Crisis* (New York: MacMillan, 1907), 285–286.

21 Good examines the ways in which missions instrumentalized medicine and education and the ways in which colonialist politics instrumentalized missions. See pp. 1–2, 5.

22 Michael Worboys, "The Colonial World as Mission and Mandate: Leprosy and Empire, 1900–1940," in *Osiris* 15(2000): 209.

23 Good, p. 3.

24 Ibid., 209–210. Worboys is quoting a British missionary working as part of the British Empire Leprosy Relief Association (BELRA) in 1927.

25 Good, p. 1, quoting the South African medical missionary James McCord.

26 John Iliffe, *The African Poor: A History* (New York: Cambridge University Press, 1987).

27 Michael Gefland, *Godly Medicine in Zimbabwe* (Harare: Memba Press, 1988), 23. Also, see Worboys, p. 209.

28 Andrew Walls, "'The Heavy Artillery of the Missionary Army': The Domestic Importance of the Nineteenth Century Medical Missionary," in *Studies in Church History, Vol. 27, The Church and Healing*, ed. William J. Shields (Oxford: Blackwell, 1982), 297–298.

29 John Mott, *The Evangelization of the World in This Generation* (New York: Student Volunteer Movement, 1905), 9.

30 Ibid., p. 15.

31 Horace Bushnell, "Science and Religion," in *Putnam's Magazine* 1, no. 3 (1868): 271. Quoted in Wendy J. Deichman Edwards, "Forging an Ideology for American Missions: Josiah Strong and

Manifest Destiny" in *North American Foreign Missions*, 1810–1914, William R. Shenk, ed. (Grand Rapids, MI: Eerdmans Publishing, 2004), 183.
32 Horace Bushnell, *Christian Nurture* (New York: Scribner, 1861), 202; 210–212.
33 Ibid., p. 183.
34 Sydney Ahlstrom, the imminent American religious historian, described Josiah Strong as "the dynamo, the revivalist, the organizer, and altogether the most irrepressible spirit of the Social Gospel movement." Quoted in Philip D. Jordan, "Josiah Strong and a Scientific Social Gospel," in *The Iliff Review* 42, no. 1 (1985): 21–31.
35 Josiah Strong, *Our Country: Its Possible Future and its Present Crisis* (New York: The Baker and Taylor Co., 1885), 163, 165, 223.
36 Quoted in Deichman Edwards, pp. 186–187.
37 The Darwin Correspondence Project has online versions of the correspondence. See www.darwinproject.ac.uk, accessed January 26, 2018). For the text of the Darwin obituary written by Fiske, see Online: http://darwin-online.org.uk/content/frameset?viewtype=text&itemID=A82&pageseq=1, accessed January 26, 2018).
38 Deichman Edwards, p. 163 (n. 1).
39 E. Berkley Tompkins, *Anti-Imperialism in the United States: The Great Debate, 1820–1920* (Philadelphia: University of Pennsylvania Press, 1970), 10–11.
40 Strong, p. 215. *Quoting John Adams, The Works of John Adams, Vol. 9* (Boston: Little, Brown & Company, 1854), 599–600. Adams recounted the event in a letter to Benjamin Rush.
41 Elizabeth Heath, "Berlin Conference of 1884–1885," in *Encyclopedia of Africa*, Henry Louis Gates, Jr. and Kwame Anthony Appiah, eds. (New York: Oxford University Press, 2010). Online: www.oxfordreference.com/view/10.1093/acref/9780195337709.001.0001/acref-9780195337709-e-0467, accessed January 26, 2018).
42 See Worboys.
43 Ibid., pp. 207–208.
44 Walter, McDougall, *Promised Land, Crusader State: The American Encounter with the World Since 1776* (New York: Houghton Mifflin, 1997). See chapter five.
45 Randall M. Packard, *A History of Global Health: Interventions into the Lives of Other People* (Baltimore: Johns Hopkins University Press, 2016), 19.
46 Ibid. Packard is quoting Mariola Espinoza, *Epidemic Invasions: Yellow Fever and the Limits of Cuban Independence* (Chicago: University of Chicago Press, 2008), 41.
47 McDougall (1997), p. 112.
48 McDougall (1997), p. 110.
49 William McKinley, *Message to Congress Requesting a Declaration of War with Spain* (letter, Washington, DC, April 11, 1898) The American Presidency Project, www.presidency.ucsb.edu/ws/?pid=103901?xid=PS_smithsonian, accessed January 26, 2018.
50 McDougall (1997), p. 111.
51 McDougall notes that a survey of 200 journals and magazines at the end of the war found sentiment in favor of annexation running three to one. McDougall (1997), pp. 112–113.
52 Thompson and Wellman, p. 16.
53 Ibid., p. 14.
54 Ibid., p. 19.
55 Roosevelt had been McKinley's Vice President. He assumed the presidency after McKinley's assassination in 1901.
56 Thompson and Wellman, p. 17.
57 Theodore Roosevelt, *Fourth Annual Message to the Senate and the House of Representatives* (speech, Washington, DC, December 6, 1804), The American Presidency Project, www.presidency.ucsb.edu/ws/index.php?pid=29545, accessed February 1, 2018.
58 S.R. Thompson and James K. Wellman, "The Social Gospel Legacy in U.S. Foreign Policy," in *Interdisciplinary Journal of Research on Religion* 7, article 6 (2011): 15.
59 McDougall (1997), p. 114.
60 Obviously, other missions took on other forms and were influenced by Christian perspectives other than the Social Gospel. Nonetheless, mainline Protestants in the progressive era – the

home of the Social Gospel movement – saw weekly attendance grow by 75% between 1895 and 1905, the years of America's brief foray into imperialism. See McDougall (1997), pp. 104–105.
61 McDougall, pp. 119–120.
62 Walter Rauschenbusch, "The Ideals of Social Reformers," in *The American Journal of Sociology* 2, no. 2 (1896): 202–203.

References

Adams, John. *The Works of John Adams, Vol. 9*. Boston: Little, Brown & Company, 1854.

Billings, John Shaw. *Public Health and Municipal Government: An Address Delivered Before the American Academy of Political and Social Science at the Art Club, Philadelphia, Jan. 14, 1891*. Philadelphia: American Academy of Political and Social Science, 1891.

Bushnell, Horace. *Christian Nurture*. New York: Scribner, 1861.

Bushnell, Horace. "Science and Religion." *Putnam's Magazine* 1, no. 3 (1868): 265–275.

Deichman Edwards, Wendy J. "Forging an Ideology for American Missions: Josiah Strong and Manifest Destiny." In *North American Foreign Missions, 1810–1914*, ed. William R. Shenk, 163–191. Grand Rapids, MI: Eerdmans Publishing, 2004.

Espinoza, Mariola. *Epidemic Invasions: Yellow Fever and the Limits of Cuban Independence*. Chicago: University of Chicago Press, 2008.

Gefland, Michael. *Godly Medicine in Zimbabwe*. Harare: Memba Press, 1988.

Good, Charles M. "Pioneer Medical Missions in Colonial Africa." *Social Science and Medicine* 32, no. 1 (1991): 1–10.

Green, Samuel G. *The Story of the Religious Tract Society for One Hundred Years*. London: The Religious Tract Society, 1899.

Griscom, John. *The Sanitary Condition of the Laboring Poor of New York*. New York: Harper & Brothers, 1845.

Hartley, Isaac Smithson. *Memorial of Robert Milham Hartley*. New York: Arno Press, 1976 (1882).

Heath, Elizabeth. "Berlin Conference of 1884–1885." In *Encyclopedia of Africa*, eds. Henry Louis Gates, Jr. and Kwame Anthony Appiah. New York: Oxford University Press, 2010. Online: www.oxfordreference.com/view/10.1093/acref/9780195337709.001.0001/acref-9780195337709-e-0467. Accessed January 26, 2018.

Hutchison, William R. *Errand to the World: American Protestant Thought and Foreign Missions*. Chicago: University of Chicago Press, 1987.

Iliffe, John. *The African Poor: A History*. New York: Cambridge University Press, 1987.

Johnson, Rossiter and John Howard Brown. *The Twentieth Century Biographical Dictionary of Notable Americans: Brief Biographies of Authors, Administrators, Clergymen, Commanders, Editors, Engineers, Jurists, Merchants, Officials, Philanthropists, Scientists, Statesmen, and Others Who Are Making American History, Volume IV: Ericsson-Gwin*. Boston: The Biographical Society, 1904.

Jordan, Philip. "Josiah Strong and A Scientific Social Gospel." *The Iliff Review* 42, no. 1 (1985): 21–31.

McKinley, William. "Message to Congress Requesting a Declaration of War with Spain." Letter, Washington, DC, April 11, 1898. The American Presidency Project. www.presidency.ucsb.edu/ws/?pid=103901?xid=PS_smithsonian. Accessed January 26, 2018.

Memoir of John Griscom, LL.D., Late Professor of Chemistry and Natural Philosophy. New York: Robert Carter and Brothers, 1859.

Mott, John. *The Evangelization of the World in This Generation*. New York: Student Volunteer Movement, 1905.

Nineteenth Annual Report of the American Tract Society. Boston: Perkins & Marvin, 1833.

Packard, Randall M. *A History of Global Health: Interventions into the Lives of Other People*. Baltimore: Johns Hopkins University Press, 2016.

Rauschenbusch, Walter. *Christianity and the Social Crisis*. New York: MacMillan, 1907.

Rauschenbusch, Walter. "The Ideals of Social Reformers." *The American Journal of Sociology* 2, no 2 (1896): 202–219.

Roosevelt, Theodore. "Fourth Annual Message to the Senate and the House of Representatives." Ppeech, Washington, DC, December 6, 1804. The American Presidency Project. www.presidency.ucsb.edu/ws/index.php?pid=29545. Accessed February 1, 2018.

Rosenberg, Charles E. and Carroll S. Rosenberg. "Pietism and the Origins of the American Public Health Movement: A Note on John H. Griscom and Robert M. Hartley." *Journal of the History of Medicine and Allied Sciences* 23:1 (January 1968): 16–35.

Strong, Josiah. *Our Country: Its Possible Future and Its Present Crisis*. New York: The Baker and Taylor Co, 1885.

Thompson, S. R. and James K. Wellman. "The Social Gospel Legacy in U.S. Foreign Policy." *Interdisciplinary Journal of Research on Religion* 7, article 6 (2011): 1–41.

Tompkins, E. Berkley. *Anti-Imperialism in the United States: The Great Debate, 1820–1920*. Philadelphia: University of Pennsylvania Press, 1970.

Twenty-Fourth Annual Report of the American Tract Society. Boston: Perkins & Marvin, 1838.

Walls, Andrew. "'The Heavy Artillery of the Missionary Army': The Domestic Importance of the Nineteenth Century Medical Missionary." In *Studies in Church History, Vol. 27, The Church and Healing*, ed. William J. Shields, 287–298. Oxford: Blackwell, 1982.

Worboys, Michael. "The Colonial World as Mission and Mandate: Leprosy and Empire, 1900–1940." *Osiris* 15 (2000): 207–218.

3 The new century begins

1900–1948

"Progressive imperialism": The Social Gospel and global health in the politics of World War I

Speaking before the annual meeting of the Health Officers of the State of New York, William Crawford Gorgas, Surgeon General of the United States Army, recounted the efforts of the United States government to address the high incidence of yellow fever through the Army's Yellow Fever Board. Gorgas had overseen the government's efforts, first in Cuba prior to and up through the Spanish-American War and later in Panama, during the construction of the Panama Canal. Gorgas began his speech by offering a litany of the devastation wrought by Yellow Fever:

> The English Army in the Windward Islands in 1794 under Sir Charles Grey, out of a total strength of 12,000 men, lost 6,000. The French Army in Santo Domingo in 1798, out of a total strength of 25,000, lost over 22,000 from yellow fever. Again in 1802 the French Army in Santo Domingo, out of a total strength of 40,000, lost 20,000. Where it prevailed it was equally fatal to civil populations. Yellow fever has many times ravaged the United States, and still more severely affected Spain. In 1798 Philadelphia, out of a population of 20,000 inhabitants who remained in the city, lost 4,000. New York City, out of a population of 50,000 in 1798, lost 2,500. New Orleans, out of a population of 100,000, lost, in 1853, 8,000 of its citizens. Spain in 1800 lost 60,000 people from yellow fever, and again in 1804, 50,000. Barcelona in 1821, of a population of 70,000, lost 16,000. Gibraltar in 1804, with a population of 10,000, lost 6,000.[1]

Gorgas recounted efforts to trace the etiology of the infection to the mosquito. The medical officers of the Army's Yellow Fever Board—Walter Reed, James Carroll, Jess Lazear, and Aristides Agramonte—worked with a Scottish-Cuban doctor named Carlos Finlay to develop a study design for testing the hypothesis that the virus was transmitted by mosquito. Gorgas spelled out the elements of the study, described the results, and interpreted their impact. He closed the speech by addressing the broader social-economic contexts that impacted health and illness:

> It is a health officer's duty to urge forward those measures in his community that will control individual diseases; but my long experience has taught me that it is still more his duty to take that broader view of life that goes to the root of bad hygiene, and do what he can to elevate the general social conditions of his community.[2]

In 1845, John Griscom and Robert Hartley had worked to address the social-economic forces that affected poor health in the tenements of New York City. Seventy years later, as he spoke to the health officers of New York State, Gorgas demonstrated the same commitment to those social factors but that commitment had been supplemented by an astounding increase in scientific knowledge. Griscom's 1845 text *The Sanitary Condition of the Laboring Poor of New York* relied on the theory of miasma or air polluted with the infectious elements of decaying matter—to account for infectious diseases such as cholera and yellow fever:

> it needs no prophetic vision to perceive, that an immense mass of offensive material, will thus be soon collected, its decomposition polluting the air, in the immediate precincts of our chambers and sitting rooms, and generating an amount of miasmatic effluvia, incalculably great and injurious. Discharge all the contents of our sinks and cispools, through sewers into the rivers, and we will avoid two of the most powerful causes of sickness and early death.[3]

Gorgas practiced medicine after the miasma theory had been discarded and doctors were aware that the very "solution" advocated by Griscom had contributed immeasurably to the spread of diseases such as yellow fever. The officers of the U.S. Army Yellow Fever Board were only able to carry out their research because of scientific discoveries in the fields of bacteriology, parasitology, incubation, microscopy, immunology, and blood typing.[4] Scientific advances had fundamentally altered the practice of medicine and had launched the field of public health. This, however, was not the only change between Griscom and Gorgas. Another fundamental change in that 70-year span between the two men is revealed in their work: Griscom was motivated (at least in part) by religious conviction to carry out his work and relied on religious structures put in place by Robert Hartley's tract missionaries to take that work to scale; Gorgas does not allude to religious conviction at all but carries out his efforts as an officer of the United States Army with the structures of the American government providing the capacity to take his work to scale.

Although the influence of the American government (and other national governments) on global health and development would grow over the course of the twentieth century, the government played almost no role in carrying out health and development initiatives as the century dawned. Public health interventions such as the yellow fever eradication efforts carried out by Gorgas and his colleagues were relegated to an aspect of military responsibility and national security. And yet, by the middle of the century, health and development initiatives—labeled as "foreign aid"—would be a key aspect of the foreign policy agendas of nations around the world. This shift was not limited to the United States. In 1938, as Europe was barreling toward the Second World War, Pasteur Vaillery-Radot, the grandson of Louis Pasteur, proclaimed:

> If peace reigns over the boundless regions, if epidemics are prevented or thwarted, if sanitary reforms can be undertaken, cities built up, and harbours opened to trade, if Europeans can live safely in hostile Africa and the Far East, if morbidity and mortality decrease in a striking way in native populations, all the transformations must be attributed to colonial medicine.[5]

In retrospect, such confidence seems willfully blind to the organized violence of colonialism, the devastation of World War I, the seismic economic quakes of the global depression of the 1930s, and the rapid approach of World War II; nonetheless, such a position was all but universal in the first decades of the twentieth century. In the United States, such confidence was grounded both in Social Gospel Protestantism and in the nation's political rhetoric.

The "progressive imperialism" articulated in in the first few years of the new century became firmly rooted in the nation over the next decade. By the start of 1910s and the administration of President Woodrow Wilson, the nation was eager to export its optimism in the steady march of progress abroad, because "the doctrine of ineluctable progress, applied to the whole human race with the United States in the vanguard, was conventional wisdom in mainstream Protestantism and peaked in the Social Gospel of Wilson's time."[6]

In May 1916, Wilson addressed the League to Enforce Peace even as Europe was mired in the first of the many "Great Wars" of the century. Wilson referenced "the Great War" before spelling out his grand plan "to see peace assume an aspect of permanence." This permanent peace was the special duty of the United States as Wilson reminded the nation's citizens that

> We are participants, whether we would or not, in the life of the world. The interests of all nations are our own also. We are partners with the rest. What affects mankind is inevitably our affair as well as the affair of the nations of Europe and of Asia. . . .
>
> So sincerely do we believe in these things that I am sure that I speak the mind and wish of the people of America when I say that the United States is willing to become a partner in any feasible association of nations formed in order to realize these objects and make them secure against violation . . . I feel

> that the world is even now upon the eve of a great consummation, when some common force will be brought into existence which shall safeguard right as the first and most fundamental interest of all peoples and all governments, when coercion shall be summoned not to the service of political ambition or selfish hostility, but to the service of a common order, a common justice, and a common peace. God grant that the dawn of that day of frank dealing and of settled peace, concord, and cooperation may be near at hand![7]

Wilson's Social Gospel allies were enthusiastic in their support of Wilson. The foremost voice to sing Wilson's praise came from the Reverend George Herron. American historian Walter McDougall describes that praise:

> None was more transfixed than George D. Herron, a leader in the Social Gospel movement who preached as fervently as his forebears that the purpose of America was to realize the Kingdom of God. Progressive reforms were purifying Americans to make them worthy of their calling. But now Wilson showed the whole world a better way. His speech, wrote Herron, was "perhaps the most pregnant utterance of a national chief in two thousand years," because he "stands for a universal politic so new, so revolutionary, so creative of a different world than ours, that few have begun to glimpse his vision or appreciate his purpose."[8]

America's Protestant leaders supported the nation's policy of neutrality in relation to the war. Protestants from across the theological and political spectrum were largely united against America's entry into the war. The Federal Council of Churches, an ecumenical network of liberal Protestants, was a strong anti-war advocate; it supported the efforts of William Jennings Bryan, Wilson's Secretary of State and a theologically conservative populist, to establish a series of peace treaties with the European powers in order to assure America's position as a neutral mediator in support of conciliation.[9] Wilson believed that America's position of neutrality would allow the country to take the lead in the creation of a just, peaceful world after the conflict had ended; he attributed this to the providence of God, stating that "Providence has deeper plans than we could possibly have laid ourselves."[10]

Neutrality might have reflected the Providence of God but the politics of humans would not allow the United States to remain above the fray. In April 1917, less than a year after Wilson's speech articulating his vision of America's role in a lasting global peace, the nation entered into the war. Even after this shift, the Federal Council of Churches remained firm in their support of Wilson:

> Thoroughly imbued with Wilsonian idealism, the Council was convinced that the war was an effort to "vindicate the principles of righteousness and the inviolability of faith between nation and nation; to safeguard the right of all

> people . . . to live their life in freedom and peace; to resist and overcome the forces that would prevent the union of the nations in a commonwealth of free peoples conscious of unity in the pursuit of ideals."[11]

The war came to an end in June of 1919, with the Treaty of Versailles representing the final set of negotiations in a ceasefire. Wilson found negotiating the concrete messiness of an armistice much more daunting than articulating the theoretical ideals of lasting global peace. In January 1918, he had laid out the principles that could lead to the end of fighting in his "Fourteen Points" speech to Congress.[12] Those points served as the basis for Wilson's position in the treaty negotiations. And it was in the process of negotiation that Wilson's idealism came into conflict with the realities of political interests. On the one hand, the representatives of the Allied Powers had little interest in idealism in light of the material and human cost of war; on the other hand, the U.S. Congress had little interest in any terms that did not protect or further America's own strategic interests. Wilson had little leverage. Wilson's allies in the United States (including the Social Gospel leaders within the Federal Council of Churches) urged Wilson to stand firm in his commitments. He did, insisting on key principles from his Fourteen Points speech that would help pave the way for the founding of the League of Nations on January 20, 1920.

For over a year, the leaders of the Federal Council of Churches waged a campaign in support of U.S. membership in the League. In 1918, the Council adopted a resolution calling the League "the political expression of the kingdom of God on earth" and presented to the U.S. Congress a petition with the signatures of over 14,000 ministers urging the support of the Treaty of Versailles.[13] Their efforts were not enough to sway the Congress. The League, indeed, had been established—but the United States was not a member. The U.S. Congress refused to support Wilson's grand ideal, even with the strong support of (Protestant) religious leaders.[14] Senator Lawrence Sherman, a Republican from Illinois, captured the mood of the Congress when he called the Covenant of the League of Nations "a revolutionary document inspired by the impossible dream of a sinless world."[15]

The Social Gospel challenged within and without

For almost 50 years, American Protestant leaders had pursued their vision of a Christianized culture. They had achieved tremendous successes in the United States in galvanizing support for a number of initiatives to address the nation's social woes on the domestic front, and they had garnered tremendous support for the cause of medical care, education, and socio-economic development in global contexts through foreign missions. The Social Gospel had been so tied to the politics of the Progressive era in American politics that the American religious historian Sydney Ahlstrom called the movement the "praying wing of progressivism."[16] When the nation's congressional representatives voted not to seek membership in the League of Nations, Social Gospelers faced defeat—an experience that had, up until then, been uncommon. That would change. Over the next two decades the façade of Protestant cohesion would crumble and critical voices against the Social Gospel goal of Christianizing the social order would grow louder. That breakdown would be seen most clearly in a crisis of confidence over a number of divisive issues within the United States itself: prohibition; immigration, eugenics, and birth control; and the teaching of evolution.

The Prohibition movement

The drinking of alcohol was widespread and growing in the British colonies and in the United States from 1720–1820. In 1720, citizens consumed on average just over two gallons of distilled spirits (whiskey, gin, etc.) per year; by 1830, the annual per capita consumption of distilled liquors had grown to over five gallons. These rates do not include consumption of fermented beverages such as wine, beer, or cider. Once these sources are added into calculations, the average American citizen is estimated to have consumed over four gallons of pure alcohol per year by 1830. Assuming that beer from that period would have approximated the alcohol content of a beer bottled today and that 12-ounce can of beer has an alcohol content of 4%, each American in 1830 would have had to drink over seven of those cans every day to achieve such numbers.[17]

American historian William Rorabaugh describes an America where alcohol flowed freely in the eighteenth and up until the mid-nineteenth century:

> Alcohol was pervasive in American society; it crossed regional, sexual, racial, and class lines. Americans drank at home and abroad, alone and together, at work and play, in fun and in earnest. They drank from the crack of dawn to the crack of dawn.[18]

Beginning in the 1830s, the social context changed drastically. American Protestantism, emboldened by the evangelistic fervor of the Second Great Awakening, launched the temperance movement and in the span of one decade, from 1830–1840, annual per capita alcohol consumption fell from just over four gallons to just under one.[19] Numerous temperance organizations were formed in the United States in the 1800s. Social Gospel leaders championed such efforts. For example, Walter Rauschenbusch supported not only voluntary temperance pledges but also legislated Prohibition.[20]

In January 1919, the United States amended its Constitution to outlaw the production, transportation, and sale of alcohol after 46 of the 48 states voted in favor ratification. For many American Protestants, the push for prohibition did not stop at the nation's borders but became a cause of foreign missions. The 1920 report of the Student Volunteer Movement for Foreign Missions[21] addressed the evils of alcohol in a perspective that also assumed a natural racial superiority of Anglo-Saxon people:

> Dr. C.H. Patton, in *The Lure of Africa*, pertinently remarks, "No race is so quickly and utterly demoralized by strong drink as the African. Self interest alone on the part of the Colonial Governments dictates that the traffic be suppressed. Yet a faltering course is allowed . . . Colonial Governors realize the destructive effects of alcohol upon native character and health, and would gladly be rid of the traffic; but financial considerations stand in the way . . . The Doctor is correct in speaking of the evil as being one of colossal magnitude—threatening the very existence of the west coast tribes. It should have the attention of the entire missionary body, the civil administrative force, and also that of the American government, which, while passing a Constitutional Amendment in favor of prohibition, within its own, should take the same high ground in its treatment of the weaker and dependent races, to whom we are sending missionaries to render medical help."[22]

The 18th Amendment to the United States Constitutions would take effect in January 1920, and all commercial alcohol production ceased with legislation supporting enforcement approved by Congress under the Volstead Act. The legislation had negative consequences. Some that were anticipated had a far deeper impact than had been anticipated but even then, most were unforeseen. An illegal, underground economy in production, transport, and sale of alcohol sprang up, leading to new crime organizations that traded not only in alcohol but also in a variety of other illegal, and often violent, activity. Without regulation, the purity of the "bathtub gin" freely dispensed at speakeasies was poor. In 1927 alone, an estimated 50,000 Americans died from consumption of alcohol tainted with impurities, and hundreds of thousands lived with permanent injuries, including blindness and paralysis. A high percentage of these poisonings came about because of the provisions of the Volstead Act, which allowed for the legal production of denatured alcohol that would be used for industrial purposes. Because this liquid was both legal and untaxed, operators of underground drinking establishments used it in the liquor they sold.[23]

Americans began to question their grand social experiment prohibiting alcohol. Many religious leaders advocated for Prohibition to remain in place, but a small, influential group of those leaders ended up playing a role in overturning the 18th Amendment even though they carried out their efforts in 1905, 15 years before Prohibition was enacted. These leaders were part of a group raising concerns about the growing national effort to enact prohibition; that group was called the Committee of Fifty for the Investigation of the Liquor Problem. In a summary of their work, the Committee's members—who included business leaders, social scientists, physicians, and clergy—wrote:

> Our members represent many different attitudes of mind toward practical methods of temperance reform . . . The problem before such a committee was that of formulating the facts on which thoughtful students of various traditions and tendencies might agree. The series of special investigations are not missionary tracts or moral appeals, but scientific studies of physical and social facts.[24]

The committee's reports represented a shift in understanding of the relationship between religious viewpoints and other sources of knowledge such as medicine, or the social or natural sciences. There was no longer an assumption of a unified vision anchored in the theological truth exemplified by American Protestantism. Obviously, the summary recommendations of the committee had little impact on popular opinion or public policy at the time the report was published since Prohibition was encoded into the Constitution 15 years later. Nonetheless, the Committee did impact alcohol prevention and treatment policy, and their research was used to build popular support for overturning prohibition.[25]

Susan Harding, a religious studies scholar, argues that the interdisciplinary work of the Committee was an important watershed for marking the end to a unified Protestant Christian ethos in the United States. She argues that

> the recommendations in the committee's volumes were largely ignored when they were published, a reflection of just how dominant the conservative Protestant "organized church forces" were at the time. But their formulation, and the coalition that came together to write them, points to the breakup of Protestant unity that was under way, even around the one issue [temperance] that had for so long brought all kinds of Protestants together.[26]

The repeal of prohibition in 1933 offered evidence that the Progressives' vision of a Christianized social order was unraveling. Debates over evolution and eugenics offered further evidence that a unified Protestant vision no longer existed.

Immigration, eugenics, and birth control

By 1910, the population of the United States had reached 92,000,000—a number larger than every country in Europe except Russia. The country had seen over 20,000,000 immigrants enter in the previous 30 years, and over one-fourth of the nation's population was foreign-born.[27] In 1885, Josiah Strong had raised the question in relation to "European peasants": "We may well ask whether this in-sweeping immigration is to foreignize us, or we are to Americanize it?"[28] Twenty-five years after Josiah Strong had first articulated his blatantly racist views, many leaders of the social gospel continued to support such rhetoric. The unabashed Americanism of the era celebrated the distinctive role of the United States to bring about lasting peace while also articulating a xenophobia of anyone who was not white, Anglo-Saxon, and Protestant. In 1899, Pope Leo condemned such displays of Americanism as a heresy that diluted the faith of European immigrants.[29]

His condemnation had little effect; by 1910, Newel Dwight Harris, the pastor of Plymouth Church in Brooklyn called for the sterilization of 10,000,000 German soldiers.[30] This racialized view of America intersected with America's budding public health movement in the field of eugenics and Social Gospel advocates were without question the strongest religious champions of the push in the nation to legalize birth control as one aspect of eugenics.

The late nineteenth century saw the emergence of the eugenics movement as new technologies provided ways to prevent pregnancy through medical devices or surgical sterilization; the movement grew rapidly through the 1930s. The eugenics movement claimed that medical technologies could improve the human population by encouraging pregnancy in some people and discouraging pregnancy or making it impossible in others. The movement's champions in public health, social work, and medicine operated under the same assumptions of the racial superiority of white, Anglo-Saxon Protestants articulated by some Social Gospel leaders such as Josiah Strong. While contraceptive technologies at the time offered one means for controlling pregnancy, the movement also advocated forced sterilization through surgery for women and men determined to be "socially inadequate." In 1914, the Director of the Eugenics Record Office and a leading eugenics advocate named Harry Laughlin drafted the "model eugenical sterilization law" that provided states with the basic framework for drafting legislation to carry out forced sterilization. When the template was created 12 states had passed sterilization laws; by 1940, 30 of the then 48 states had passed such laws crafted from Laughlin's template. In 1939, the Reichstag in Germany referred to the model law in crafting its own legislations, the Law for the Prevention of Hereditarily Diseased Offspring.[31]

The law reflected general consensus among leaders of the eugenics movement and defined the "socially inadequate classes" as follows:

> The socially inadequate classes, regardless of etiology or prognosis, are the following: 1) feeble-minded; 2) insane . . .; 3) Criminalistic . . .; 4) Epileptic; 5) Inebriate . . .; 6) Diseased . . .; 7) Blind . . .; 8) Deaf . . .; 9) Deformed . . .; and 10) Dependent.

The law then laid out the legal definition of a cacogenic person—a potential parent of a socially inadequate offspring—who could be subject to forced sterilization:

> A potential parent of socially inadequate offspring is a person, who, regardless of his or her own physical, physiological, or psychological personality, and of the nature of the germ-plasm of such person's co-parent, is a potential parent at least one fourth of whose possible offspring, because of the certain inheritance from said parent of one or more inferior or degenerate physical, physiological, or psychological qualities would, on the average, according to the demonstrated laws of heredity, most probably function as socially inadequate person; or at least one-half of whose possible offspring would receive from said parent and carry in the germ-plasm but would not necessarily show in the personality, the genes or genes-complex for one or more inferior or degenerate physical, physiological, or psychological qualities, the appearance of which quality would cause the possessor thereof to function as a socially inadequate person under the normal environment of the state.[32]

The leaders of the eugenics movement championed an unabashed and uncritical vision of racial supremacy. Those leaders succeeded in passing laws that mandated sterilization for those deemed inadequate. A number of Jewish and Protestant Christian leaders were counted among those champions; Roman Catholic moral theology on contraception made such support out of the question for Roman Catholic clergy. Sociologists Melinda J. Wilde and Sabrina Danielson examined the written materials of 28 different religious bodies from 1929–1931—25 different Protestant denominations, Roman Catholicism, Conservative Judaism, and Reform Judaism—and identified nine of those denominations as the early supporters of contraceptives. All nine had two distinctive characteristics that were not found among the other nineteen: 1) all were supporters of social gospel initiatives, and 2) all supported the concept of race suicide—"the belief that white Anglo-Saxon Protestants were being outbred by southern and eastern European immigrants."[33] Those denominations were (see Table 3.1):

Table 3.1 Religious bodies supportive of birth control on the basis of eugenics in 1928 and the names of those bodies today

Religious body name (1929)	*Religious body name (2018)*
1. Society of Friends (Quakers)	1. Society of Friends (Quakers)
2. Reform Judaism	2. Reform Judaism
3. Universalist Church	3. Unitarian Universalist Association*
4. American Unitarian Association	
5. Methodist Episcopal Church	4. United Methodist Church
6. Congregational Churches	5. United Church of Christ
7. Christian Church	6. Christian Church, Disciples of Christ
8. Presbyterian Church in the USA	7. Presbyterian Church in the USA
9. Protestant Episcopal Church	8. Protestant Episcopal Church in the USA

* The Universalist Church and the American Unitarian Association merged into a single denomination—the Unitarian Universalist Association—in 1961.

These nine religious bodies provided the religious foundation for a racialized vision of birth control; they legitimated birth control, organized social support, and made established formal positions in favor of liberalization. The American Eugenics Society, had a specific initiative—the Committee for Cooperation with Clergymen—aimed at recruiting religious leaders as "eugenic apostles" (i.e., spokespersons) for the movement. Columns in the Society's journal *Eugenics* were penned by religious leaders who supported birth control, involuntary sterilization, and limited immigration in regard to southern and eastern Europeans while urging white, Anglo-Saxon Protestants to create an ideal family of at least four children.[34] It is important to note that not all Social Gospel champions supported this vision of racialized birth control. Wilde and Danielson identify nine other religious bodies[35] which supported the Social Gospel but did not support the concept of race suicide and therefore did not publicly advocate for liberalization of birth control. American Protestantism was clearly a force in the racialized and racist ideas so prevalent in American society in the early decades of the twentieth century. The question remains, however: did such views influence foreign missions or governments' foreign policy? In fact, they did.

Colonial administrators in the British colonies on the African continent during the interwar years carried out various epidemiological surveillance interventions to assess levels of sterility and male fertility. The colonies were "undergoing a crisis of biological reproduction—they were simply not reproducing themselves at a sufficient rate to ensure the economic viability of the colonies."[36] The Secretary of State for the Colonies published a circular to the colonial governors in 1930 that referenced these concerns:

> It has recently been represented to me that the numbers of the native population in many parts of the Empire is stationary, if not actually on the decrease, and that the general level of their physique is considerably below standard . . . It has been suggested to me that, in many places, low health standards and slow increase in population may in large measure be attributed to the prevalence of certain native customs which are directly repugnant to European ideas of hygiene and medical knowledge.[37]

Medical officials identified two inter-related causes for this precipitous drop in birth rates: the absence of "better males" who could keep the wanton sexuality of women in check, and cultural norms that lowered fertility by hindering male virility and leaving women with little power to challenge dehumanizing practices.[38]

American global medical missions also took up the issue of eugenics. The most direct example of this can be seen in the medical mission efforts of John Henry Kellogg, a medical doctor and Seventh Day Adventist missionary who founded the American Medical Missionary Board in 1891 and the American Medical Missionary College in 1895 to support global medical missions. In 1914, Kellogg disbanded the Board as he shifted his focus from the education and support of medical missions to eugenics efforts globally. The Board formally changed its name to the Race Betterment Foundation. In the final issue of the journal *The Medical Missionary* that Kellogg published, he wrote:

> Medical mission work has come to be recognized as an integral and essential feature of evangelistic effort. The example of our Saviour in uniting the healing of the body with the restoration of the soul in one Gospel is now understood by our great missionary bodies.
>
> Recently the name of our association was changed from The American Medical Missionary Association to the Race Betterment Foundation. This change indicates the direction which our principal efforts are to take for the present. We do not wish to imply that we relinquish our interest in the noble efforts of missionaries in foreign lands.[39]

The same month, he publicized the Foundation in another journal he published entitled *Good Health* ("The Oldest Health Magazine in America"):

> With half the human race engaged in the bloodiest war of all time, the world has before it a most striking example of the need of race betterment, and of the imminent danger of race deterioration . . . The greater loss, one which must extend to all succeeding generations and with ever increasing proportions, is the cutting off of these lines of vigorous, healthy human stock, an absolutely appalling and irreparable loss. That war is a most active factor in race degeneracy, Dr. David Starr Jordan has ably pointed out. The European war is killing off, not sick men or weaklings, which are the chief victims of epidemic and endemic scourges, but the finest and healthiest, the fittest for propagating the race . . . More than ever, efforts toward race betterment are needed—are, indeed, imperative . . . The race betterment movement which was inaugurated at Battle Creek last January aims to coordinate and unify so far as possible all the forces which are working for the physical upbuilding of men and the development of a new race of human thoroughbreds.[40]

Evolution

William Jennings Bryan, "The Great Commoner," was a leading political and cultural figure in America in the late nineteenth and early twentieth century. From 1891–1895, he served the first district of the state of Nebraska in the U.S. Congress as a member of the House of Representatives. From 1913–1915, he served as the United States Secretary of State under President Woodrow Wilson, resigning over Wilson's decision to take the nation into World War I. Bryan was a Presidential nominee for President in 1908 but lost to William Howard Taft.

On many issues, Bryan aligned with Social Gospel advocates. He was deeply committed to workers' rights; use of taxation to lessen economic disparities; government aid to farmers, public ownership of the railroads, telephone, and telegraph; government guarantee of bank deposits; women's suffrage; federal departments of education and health; temperance; a "benevolent imperialism" as a new aspect of American foreign policy; and anti-war advocacy.[41] Bryan was a devout Christian who framed all of his political and policy positions as an expression of his faith:

> I know what democracy means—it is a religion, and when you hear a good democratic speech it is so much like a sermon that you can hardly tell the difference between them. A good sermon is built upon the ten commandments, the sermon on the mount, and the eleventh commandment: "Thou shalt love thy neighbor as thyself." And a good democratic speech is built upon the doctrine of human brotherhood, equal rights, and self government.[42]

But there were two issues on which Bryan differed when compared to many Social Gospel leaders: eugenics and evolution.

For 12 days in 1925, Americans were mesmerized by the trial proceedings being carried out in the courtroom of the small town of Dayton, Tennessee. John Thomas Scopes, the football coach and substitute teacher at the local high school, was on trial for violating a law passed by the state legislature only four months before that outlawed the teaching of evolutionary theory in the state's schools. Bryan agreed to serve as part of the prosecuting team, which turned the trial into a national spectacle that newspapers around the country termed "the trial of the century." The prosecuting attorney, Clarence Darrow, was dismissive of Bryan and his ideas, stating that "I made up my mind to show the country what an ignoramus he was, and I succeeded."[43] After one hour of deliberation, the jury found Scopes guilty; Darrow and national civil rights organizations were heartened by the ruling because the verdict would allow for appeal to higher courts and build public support for their position that scientific theory rather than biblical narrative should serve as the basis for teaching biology. Five days after the verdict, Bryan unexpectedly died, still living in the house he had rented for the duration of the trial in Dayton. The famous newspaper columnist H.L. Mencken had covered the entire trial for *The Baltimore Sun*. On the day of Bryan's death, the paper published the obituary penned by Mencken, which read in part:

> Bryan was a vulgar and common man, a cad undiluted. He was ignorant, bigoted, self-seeking, blatant and dishonest. His career brought him into contact with the finest men of his time; he preferred the company of rustic ignoramuses. It was hard to believe, watching him at Dayton, that he had traveled, that he had been received in civilized societies, that he had been a high officer of state. He seemed only a poor clod like those around him, deluded

> by a childish theology, full of an almost pathological hatred of all learning, all human dignity, all beauty, all fine and noble things. He was a peasant come home to the dung-pile. Imagine a gentleman, and you have imagined everything that he was not.

Mencken, one might surmise, was no fan. In his support of Tennessee's prohibition on teaching evolution, Bryan cemented a perception in American popular culture of a mean-spirited, close-minded, incurious, dogmatic Christian fundamentalist, and the Scopes Monkey Trial, as the trial came to be known, was seen as a seminal moment in the battle between science and religious fundamentalism—a battle that has continued on until this day. On one side, according to this popular perception, were the clear-eyed champions of science and on the other were religious zealots who refused to accept scientific fact and chose to cling to superstition based on simplistic and willfully ignorant readings of scripture.[44] But such sharp divisions are much less clear in reality.

Matthew Tontonoz, a biologist and social historian, argues that the Bryan was less a fundamentalist creationist than a devout but fair-minded Christian who rejected Darwinism because it conflicted with the social and political views that he as a Christian could not abide, namely social Darwinism and eugenics. In his analysis of Bryan's closing arguments,[45] Tontonoz notes that Bryan raised no objection to evolutionary theory based on scientific or religious grounds and did not articulate the state's position using religious claims. Rather, Bryan focused on the ways in which evolutionary theory underwrote a Social Darwinism that he found both immoral and cruel by constructing harsh social theories that justified the dismantling of social support programs in the interest of the "survival of the fittest."

The textbook used in Tennessee to teach evolutionary theory also taught eugenics as a natural corollary to Darwin's ideas. Historian Andrew Nolan has argued that the book

> embedded the combination of scientific knowledge, public health management and state reforms within a framework of ideological assumptions about human races and civilizations. The textbook provided a taxonomy of human racial development for students that encompassed "five races or variety of man, each very different from the other in instincts, social customs, and, to an extent, in structure." Hunter's description of human varieties bore strong similarities to the ascending ladder of races portrayed in lists and portraits in the late 1800s and early 1900s.[46]

In short, Bryan's key concern wasn't Biblical (though he did have theological reservations)—it was in a science that failed to mirror his belief in moral progressivism. Bryan's death, however, proved a more telling symbol for interpretations of the trial that emerged over the next several decades. These accounts described the event as a triumph for a vision of Progressive reform led by scientific men who would help free modern citizens from the strictures of conservative Christian dogmatism. And these interpretations have since predominated whenever the trial is discussed.

Church historian Janet Fishburn has argued that both theologically liberal and theologically conservative Christians in the early twentieth century were committed to social reform. While Social Gospel champions such as Rauschenbusch championed

> a theology in which the gospel is understood as social in its very nature [and that] social institutions, societies, and nations are capable of the kind of radical change—or conversion—usually associated only with individuals during the revivals or "awakenings" of the first half of the nineteenth century. What Rauschenbusch often failed to mention was the extent to which the missionary movement at home and abroad had been concerned with social reform.[47]

Fishburn's claim does not fit with our present-day delineations of liberal and conservative in either a political or a theological sense. Nonetheless, her claim does fit with the evidence in regard to eugenics, evolution, and prohibition. In the first decades of the 1920s, American Protestantism enjoyed tremendous social power not only to influence public opinion but also to help set government priorities and policies. In the same decades, however, American Protestantism began to splinter. This is not to say that the theological positions of Episcopalians in New York and Baptists in Nebraska had ever been the same; rather, it points to evidence that Protestants had established shared commitments in the midst of their differences—one of those being a shared commitment to foreign missions—which had allowed for some degree of unity up until the 1920s. This unity began to splinter in the early 1900s, even as the movement could wield tremendous social power.

In the aftermath of the First World War and the economic hardships experienced as the nation into the Great Depression in the 1930s, Protestant unity devolved into doctrinal suspicion and the advocates of the Social Gospel saw their congregations enter into a decline for the first time in almost a century. Under such circumstances, it is surprising then to realize that Social Gospelers' attempts to Christianize the social order would come to impact American and international policies in ways they could not have imagined.

The time period in which the tenets of the Social Gospel were articulated is also the same period in which one of America's wealthiest families carried out programs marked by religious piety and bankrolled with their own money that have had a lasting impact on global health and development practice up to the present. The Rockefeller family influenced liberal Protestantism, public health research, global health practice, and American politics in a way no other family has.

The Social Gospel embodied in the Rockefellers

He was a faithful leader at Cleveland's Euclid Avenue Baptist Church in the early 1900s, giving generously in support of the church's ministries and its operating budget. Though he was a hard-working businessman, religious practice in the form of pietistic devotion to this church community grounded his life. He taught Sunday School for decades and even served as Superintendent for a time. Many of his Saturday afternoons consisted of sweeping the chapel floors, replacing candles in the sconces, or stacking the stove in the corner (the only source of heat in the building) with wood—all in preparation for the next day's worship. He always dressed in coat and tie, not only at church but during the work week; his wife and children dressed similarly in clothes that were respectable but not ostentatious and he stated that they would always "wear their Sunday clothes to work and school as a sign of Christian pride."[48] He and his family always sat in the same ninth-row pew. Euclid Avenue was a working-class congregation where "all but a half-dozen of the families were of limited means."[49] His children each presented their offerings to the church on a weekly basis, and their father was clear that the money "will be earned by the sweat of their brows, pulling weeds and the like."[50] As a young adult, he went for a period of time without any place to live and walked the streets of Cleveland looking for work. He often referred to that time in his life when teaching Sunday School, expressing gratitude for finding a part-time job as bookkeeper for a dock warehouse. An artifact from that job—an account ledger—took on religious significance for him:

> The little book is most significant. No wonder, as he once told his Sunday-school class, holding up [the ledger] to their attentive eyes: "You could not get that book from me for all the modern ledgers in New York, nor for all that they would bring. It almost brings tears to my eyes when I read over this little book, and it fills me with a sense of gratitude I cannot express."[51]

This man was the picture of Protestant piety and propriety—an object lesson on the importance of hard work, fiscal restraint, and familial commitments to faithful devotion to Jesus Christ. He was also the richest man in the world at the time—someone whose personal wealth equaled about two percent of the total annual economic output of the United States and someone whose wealth today would equal about $280,000,000,000, or about three times the wealth controlled by Bill Gates.[52] He was John D. Rockefeller, Sr., the founder of Standard Oil Company.

The story of this man, his son John Jr., and grandson Nelson offers a clear case study of Social Gospel ideals being taken up in the structures of government and civil society from 1900 to 1980. The senior Rockefeller's gifts to colleges and universities across the country (most of them founded and supported by Baptists) is well-documented. Without question, the gift that is best known was his initial gift of $600,000 (the present-day value would be over $25,000,000) toward the founding of the University of Chicago in 1890.[53] While that gift is significant, it was by no means the first.[54] That distinction goes to Kenyon College, which was the recipient of a $5.00 donation from Rockefeller in 1864. Far more substantial gifts to various schools followed. Rockefeller gave $22,500 to Denison University (founded by Baptists in Granville, Ohio) in five separate donations between 1868 and 1882. He gave a small donation to Chicago University, the predecessor to the university he later helped endow.[55]

Rockefeller support was essential for establishing a number of colleges for African-Americans and Native Americans in the United States. A donation to A.C. Bacone in 1881 led to the founding of Bacone College, a Baptist undergraduate institution for Native Americans in Oklahoma. An 1862 donation to Sophia Packard and Harriet Giles allowed the Atlanta Female Seminary to establish its own campus; the school's trustees changed the name of the college to Spelman, the maiden surname of Mrs. Rockefeller, in honor of her abolitionist family whose home was a stop on the Underground Railroad.[56] Rockefeller provided a series of donations to the Atlanta Baptist Seminary, including a donation in support of its move from Augusta, Georgia, to Atlanta that provided the land for the school's campus; the seminary was renamed for Henry L. Morehouse, who was Executive Secretary of the American Baptist Home Mission Society. Today, Spelman and Morehouse anchor the Atlanta University Center, a consortium of historically black colleges just west of downtown Atlanta.[57]

The University of Chicago received the personal $600,000 donation from Rockefeller (his total donations to the university would eventually total approximately $35,000,000, or over $875,000,000 today);[58] it also received financial support from the American Baptist Education Society, an official ministry office of the American Baptist denomination. In fact, the office only existed because of Rockefeller's financial support.[59] From 1890 to 1914, the Society, with Rockefeller as the only significant contributor paid out over $800,000 to 34 different schools.[60] The relationship between Rockefeller and the Society established a precedent the family built on of contributing to an independent philanthropic entity which would reflect the family's commitments and priorities. Upon the death of John D. Rockefeller, Sr. in 1937, the *New York Times* reported that he had donated over $530,000,000 through four foundations: the Rockefeller Institute for Medical Research, the Rockefeller Foundation, the Laura Spelman Rockefeller Memorial, and the General Education Board (which was the non-religious, independent entity that grew out of the American Baptist Education Society).[61]

John D. Rockefeller, Jr. continued his father's legacy of religious piety and charitable giving. He was a faithful member of Park Avenue Baptist Church in Manhattan until he decided to establish and endow The Riverside Church, a nondenominational

Protestant congregation in the upper west side Manhattan neighborhood of Morningside Heights in 1925.[62] Riverside became the guardian of the Social Gospel tradition from the moment it was founded up to the present. The stained glass and statuary in the church memorialized in its statues and stained glass honor Charles Darwin, Mohammed, Buddha, Albert Einstein, Abraham Lincoln, and Booker T. Washington along with Biblical and religious figures.[63] Its founding pastor, Harry Emerson Fosdick, "carried the social gospel banner into the midcentury."[64] Fosdick believed that Riverside Church would

> help the younger generation discover its divine vocation and say, "Here I am, send me. If wherever soldiers of the common good are fighting for a more decent international life and a juster industry, they should feel behind them the support this church, which . . . has kept its conviction clear that a major part of Christianity is the application of the principles of Jesus to the social life, and that no industrial or international question is settled until it is settled Christianly."[65]

In the 1920s, Rockefeller provided over $1,000,000 to the Union Theological Seminary in the City of New York, the Protestant Seminary most closely associated with the Social Gospel.[66] Under the auspices of the Foundation and the General Education Board, Rockefeller funded theological education for historically black seminaries and minority seminarians, including donations to the Interdenominational Theological Center, the largest historically black seminary in the world,[67] and special endowments to the Forum for Theological Education to provide scholarship support for racial and ethnic minority communities.[68]

But John D. Rockefeller, Jr. did not limit his attention or his charitable giving to religious institutions. For that matter, neither did his father. From its founding, the Rockefeller Foundation supported a variety of international health initiatives. One of the first initiatives following the founding of the Foundation in 1913 was the funding of the Chinese Medical Board whose goal was to establish two medical schools in China by 1920 with another to follow thereafter. To carry out this objective, the Foundation initially relied on the medical missionaries already established in the country:

> The decision to establish two medical centers, the one at Peking and the other at Shanghai, will lay a base line along the coast from which other centers may be established at a later date under the auspices of the Foundation, through missionary initiative, or as government enterprises . . . The Commissioners [of the Rockefeller Foundation] referred to are quoted as saying in effect to missionary educators, 'We are thinking of the interests of China as a whole . . . Will you join us and make a happy combination, and be as keen on Christianity as we are on medical science? . . . The Foundation has the financial resources

> with which to do in laboratory, class room, and hospital what no one Board, nor half a dozen Boards with their obligations, could possibly do . . . Scientifically qualified men are required, but Christian men of equal qualifications are preferred. Let men offer for such service, secure the best preparation there is to be had, and . . . train a body of Chinese physicians and surgeons who can in turn not only man mission and government hospitals, but become the influential factors for moral purity and religious life in the institutions of the country.[69]

At the time of its inception, the Rockefeller Foundation established partnerships with foreign medical mission organizations to carry out its work. By the early 1930s, public health had become a priority for the Foundation. The International Health Commission was established by the Foundation in 1913 (the name was changed to the International Health Board in 1916 and the International Health Division in 1927), the year the Foundation was founded. This body would become "the most powerful and influential international health organization during the first half of the twentieth century."[70] The International Health Division of the Rockefeller Foundation exercised tremendous influence within the League of Nations Health Organization (LNHO), the predecessor body to the World Health Organization. The LNHO faced chronic budget shortfalls during the global economic depression of the 1930s and the Foundation provided over a third of its total budget. In return, the Foundation influenced priorities within the LNHO, establishing a focus on scientific and organizational issues and minimizing social and economic factors on poor health.[71]

The Foundation focused on building public health education globally. In the United States, it endowed the School of Hygiene and Public Health at Johns Hopkins University in 1918, and in1921, it endowed both the School of Public Health at Harvard and the School of Public Health at the University of Michigan.[72] Globally, the Foundation eventually funded the London School ofTropical Medicine and Hygiene and 20 other schools or programs of public health across the globe over the next two decades.[73]

After the end of World War II, the Rockefellers played key roles in establishing both religious and governmental global health and development institutions. The Foundation funded the establishment of the Ecumenical Institute of the World Council of Churches in 1946, a global Protestant Christian body that has been active on health and development programs and advocacy for over 70 years.[74] John D. Rockefeller, Jr. purchased 17 acres on the east side of Manhattan for $8.5 million in 1946 and then donated the land to serve as the headquarters of the newly-formed United Nations.[75] Finally, in 1959, John D. Rockefeller, Jr. provided the land and funds for building the Interchurch Center of the National Council of Churches (NCC) on Manhattan's upper west side just south of Riverside Church and Union Theological Seminary. Twenty thousand people lined the streets, and President Dwight Eisenhower delivered the opening address at the opening of the center.[76]

The NCC wielded a great deal of social and political power at the time by articulating the social policy positions of mainline Protestant denominations on domestic and global issues and working with the World Council of Churches in Geneva. Mainline denominations also housed the headquarters of their respective offices in domestic and foreign missions, social action, and development in the Interchurch Center. Finally, the Rockefeller Foundation was influential in setting the priorities of various agencies within the United Nations through its direct contributions to the body and by providing grant funding to those agencies for specific programs.[77]

The last example of the Rockefellers' influence is seen in the career of Nelson Rockefeller, son of John D. Rockefeller, Jr. Nelson did not remain involved in the business interests of his father and grandfather (though he helped to manage the fortune made off of those interests) but opted for a career in government, serving as Assistant Secretary of State for American Affairs for President Roosevelt during World War II and President Truman after the war; Undersecretary of the Department of Health, Education, and Welfare under President Eisenhower; Governor of New York State; and Vice President to President Ford. The following description of Nelson Rockefeller's efforts to implement health and development initiatives in Latin America as part of the work of the U.S. State Department during World War II demonstrates the extent to which the Social Gospel legacy of the generations before him had become inculcated into his work in the government's foreign policy initiatives:

> The attempt to make permanent improvements in the health of other peoples represented for [Nelson] Rockefeller a unique conjunction of national and family history. The types of aid programs he proposed had originated with Christian missionaries in the late nineteenth century. These individuals preached the gospel of modem science and medicine as well as that of Christ. John D. Rockefeller, Sr., the greatest supporter of missionaries in his generation, expanded and secularized this tradition with the creation of the Rockefeller Foundation, the first significant private nonsectarian institution to provide assistance in medicine and public health to developing nations. His grandson played a prominent role in making that tradition an accepted part of the U.S. foreign policy establishment.[78]

Some background into these Latin American initiatives offers insight into the ways in which the Rockefeller family influenced American foreign policy.

In the course of the Second World War, the United States realized that government and civil society perceptions in countries in Central and South America were causes of concern. Germany had established a foothold in the French colonies of West Africa with the establishment of the Vichy government in France. Analysts in the U.S. believed that German aircraft capabilities from the western reaches of the African continent put them in striking range of northeastern Brazil; were the Nazis to establish a base there, the Panama Canal in Central America would be at risk. Economic factors aligned with this military scenario against the United States; countries in Central and South America had lost their trading partners in Europe—the primary engines of the nations' economies—because of the war and there were some factions in the countries pushing for a German victory.

Committed to a united Western Hemisphere under the leadership of the United States, President Roosevelt gave Rockefeller as Coordinator for American Affairs tremendous authority to coordinate the Institute for Inter-American Affairs (IIAA) in Latin America. Initially, the scope of the Institute was rather limited: provide economic incentives through direct infrastructure investments; establish trade deals between the United States and countries in the region; formulate American propaganda to counter pro-Nazi views in the region; and implement cultural exchange initiatives.

Rockefeller expanded the role of the IIAA while simultaneously answering concerns that the initiative was draining off financial and personnel resources that could better be used directly in the European or Pacific theatres of the war. He suggested that the American military furnish the IIAA with the locations of likely bases as part of their strategic planning to push back against Nazi efforts in the region should they coalesce. In response, the IIAA would coordinate infrastructure building of hospitals, sanitation and water systems, communication facilities, and transportation networks. Some of the identified strategic sites were located in areas with poor health infrastructure and high disease incidence. Rockefeller set out not only to build infrastructure but also to improve the health of the people in those locations.

As part of those efforts, the IIAA provided health education through radio broadcasts, print media, and movies. Walt Disney created animated shorts on such topics as infant care, proper precautions against insects that might transmit diseases, and the hazards of contaminated water. The most popular was *Winged Scourge*,[79] which used the Seven Dwarfs to teach about transmission of malaria. Another, *Defense Against Invasion*, taught about the science behind vaccination using the metaphor of disease as invading enemy and vaccination as the weapon to ward off the menacing threat.[80]

Many in the War Department wondered how the work of the IIAA, which included production of cartoons to relay health information, contributed to the country's efforts to defeat the Axis Powers, In Congressional testimony, General George Dunham, a member of the U.S. Army Medical Corps who had been named Chief Physician in the European theater before being selected to head the public health efforts of the IAA, joined Rockefeller in front of the House Appropriations

Committee in 1943 to testify that these efforts had a direct connection to the nation's defense:

MR. O'NEAL: [a Congressional representative]: Is there is a direct relationship between the location of every dispensary [in support of malaria control] and the Allied war needs?
GENERAL DUNHAM: Every place where there is need.
MR. O'NEAL: But you have no dispensaries for the general health of the community.
GENERAL DUNHAM: Oh yes; we have, and must have, to fulfill our cooperative agreements with those countries.
MR. O'NEAL: What is the underlying reason for that?
GENERAL DUNHAM: To improve the general public health.
MR. O'NEAL: Without any relationship to the war effort?
GENERAL DUNHAM: It has a general relationship.
MR. O'NEAL: To have a stronger Allied country, but you cannot relate it specifically to any direct contribution to the war effort except the general effect.
GENERAL DUNHAM: We do that. The public health cannot be restricted to one area. That sort of development could be applied to any part of the world.
MR. O'NEAL: Would you say everything we have done there has something directly to do with the war effort?
MR. ROCKEFELLER: Absolutely.[81]

The project continued through the war, but many in the State Department and the War Department thought it a waste of time and resources. There seemed little chance that the work of the IIAA would continue after the war but Rockefeller was determined. In 1944, he was promoted to Assistant Secretary of State and in that position, he wrote President Roosevelt a memorandum outlining his approach to Latin American engagement, detailing long-tern cooperation in "public health, nutrition and food supply, education, science, culture, information, transportation, economic development and modernization of agriculture." Roosevelt strongly backed the proposal, swayed by Rockefeller's reasoning that:

> These are the basic factors which contribute to the development and dignity of the individual, a rising standard of living and growth of democracy. Only in this way can we hope to have economic, social, and political stability among the nations of this Hemisphere—without which we can never realize the permanent unity of the Americas.[82]

Roosevelt died on April 12, 1945 before acting on the memo and before seeing Germany's surrender less than a month later. His vice-president, Harry S. Truman, assumed the presidency. With support from ambassadors in Latin America, the IIAA project was extended for three years but was to be shuttered in 1950. It likely would have been, except for the efforts of a speechwriter in the new administration of President Truman named Benjamin Hardy. Hardy had worked for Rockefeller in carrying out IIAA efforts in Brazil and he included a reference to the project in Truman's inauguration speech but the State Department removed it. Hardy called a colleague at the White House and left a memorandum outlining the program. Truman read the memorandum and liked the idea; he sent the speech back to the State Department for revision, instructing that the principles included in the outline memorandum be included.

On January 20, 1949, Harry Truman was re-inaugurated as the 33rd President of the United States. His inauguration speech outlined four priorities of his administration. The fourth point related to foreign affairs and international development:

> Fourth, we must embark on a bold new program for making the benefits of our scientific advances and industrial progress available for the improvement and growth of underdeveloped areas. More than half the people of the world are living in conditions approaching misery. Their food is inadequate. They are victims of disease. Their economic life is primitive and stagnant. Their poverty is a handicap and a threat both to them and to more prosperous areas.
>
> For the first time in history, humanity posesses [*sic*] the knowledge and skill to relieve suffering of these people. The United States is pre-eminent among nations in the development of industrial and scientific techniques. The material resources which we can afford to use for assistance of other peoples are limited. But our imponderable resources in technical knowledge are constantly growing and are inexhaustible.
>
> I believe that we should make available to peace-loving peoples the benefits of our store of technical knowledge in order to help them realize their aspirations for a better life. And, in cooperation with other nations, we should foster capital investment in areas needing development.
>
> Our aim should be to help the free peoples of the world, through their own efforts, to produce more food, more clothing, more materials for housing, and more mechanical power to lighten their burdens. We invite other countries to pool their technological resources in this undertaking. Their contributions will be warmly welcomed. This should be a cooperative enterprise in which all nations work together through the United Nations and its specialized agencies whenever practicable. It must be a worldwide effort for the achievement of peace, plenty, and freedom.[83]

Truman's speech became known as the "Point Four" speech. It laid out for the first time America's approach to health and development aid as an aspect of the nation's overall foreign policy. Point Four led to the eventual creation of the U.S. Agency for International Development. Nelson Rockefeller's efforts through the IIAA were a catalyst for embedding international health and development programs as part of the nation's foreign policy strategy.

Across three generations and through diverse mechanisms such as personal donations, foundation activities, and political leadership, the Rockefellers played a key role in transitioning the Social Gospel from a theological vision articulated by a group of influential Protestant leaders at the end of the nineteenth century to some of the central principles of U.S. and global governmental bodies. They embody, in other words, an effort to transfer the empire of the world from a specifically Christian framework into a secular context. Their efforts reflect the ways in which a distinctly American and Christian notion of a Christianized social order became secularized and internationalized. The next chapter develops this idea of a secularized Christianity being taken up in a variety of global health and development efforts.

Notes

1 William Gorgas, "Tropical Sanitation in its Relation to General Sanitation," in *The Journal of the American Medical Association* 65, no. 26 (1915): 2208.

2 Ibid., p. 2009.

3 John Griscom, *The Sanitary Condition of the Laboring Poor of New York* (New York: Harper & Brothers, 1845), 52.

4 Randall M. Packard, *A History of Global Health: Interventions into the Lives of Other People* (Baltimore: Johns Hopkins University Press, 2016), 25.

5 Michael Worboys, "The Colonial World as Mission and Mandate: Leprosy and Empire, 1900–1940," in *Osiris* 15 (2000): 211.

6 S.R. Thompson and James K. Wellman, "The Social Gospel Legacy in U.S. Foreign Policy," in *Interdisciplinary Journal of Research on Religion* 7, article 6 (2011): 25.

7 Woodrow Wilson, *Address Delivered to the First Annual Assemblage of the League to Enforce Peace: 'American Principles,'* (speech, Washington, DC, May 27, 1916), The American Presidency Project, www.presidency.ucsb.edu/ws/?pid=65391, accessed February 4, 2108.

8 Walter McDougall, *Promised Land: Crusader State: The American Encounter with the World Since 1776* (New York: Houghton Mifflin, 1997), 123.

9 Ralph L. Pearson, "Internationalizing the Social Gospel: The Federal Council of Churches and European Protestantism, 1914–1925," in *Historical Magazine of the Protestant Episcopal Church* 52, no. 3 (1983): 276–277.

10 Thompson and Wellman, p. 21.

11 Ibid., p. 279.

12 Woodrow Wilson, "Address to a Joint Session of Congress on the Conditions for Peace," (speech, Washington, DC, January 8, 1918), The American Presidency Project, www.presidency.ucsb.edu/ws/index.php?pid=65405&st=&st1=, accessed February 5, 2018

13 Pearson, p. 280.

14 For background on the complexities of these various forces on Wilson's ideals, see Walter McDougall, *Promised Land: Crusader State: The American Encounter with the World Since 1776* (New York: Houghton Mifflin, 1997), chapter six, "Wilsonianism, or Liberal Internationalism."

15 See McDougall (1997), p. 145.

16 Janet F. Fishburn, "The Social Gospel as Missionary Ideology," in *North American Foreign Missions, 1810–1914*, William R. Shenk, ed. (Grand Rapids, MI: Eerdmans Publishing, 2004), 220.

17 W. J. Rorabaugh, *The Alcoholic Republic: An American Tradition* (New York: Oxford University Press, 1979), 7–8.

18 Ibid., pp. 20–21.

19 Ibid., p. 7
20 Susan Harding, "American Protestant Moralism and the Secular Imagination: From Temperance to the Moral Majority," in *Social Research* 76, no. 4 (Winter 2009): 1294.
21 Student missionary organizations generated and mobilized tremendous capacities in carrying out mission work. In 1920, 2,700 university students volunteered for extended time on the foreign mission field at the Foreign Mission Conference of North America. See Robert T. Handy, "The American Religious Depression, 1925–1935," in *Church History* 29, no. 1 (1960): 5.
22 Walter R. Lambuth, *Medical Missions: The Two-fold Task* (New York: Student Volunteer Movement for Foreign Missions, 1920), 21–22.
23 Edward Behr, *Prohibition: Fifteen Years that Changed America* (New York: Arcade Publishing, 1996), 221–222.
24 Francis Peabody, "Introduction," in *The Liquor Problem: A Summary of Investigations Conducted by The Committee of Fifty* (New York: Houghton, Mifflin, and Company, 1905), 7–8.
25 For information on the Committee's influence on alcohol policy and on overturning the 18th Amendment, see Holland Webb, "Temperance Movements and Prohibition," in *International Social Science Review* 74, no. 1/2 (1999): 61–69. Also, see Harry Gene Levine, "The Committee of Fifty and the Origins of Alcohol Control," in *Journal of Drug Issues* 13, no. 1 (1983): 95–116.
26 Harding, p. 1297.
27 McDougall (1997), pp. 102–103.
28 Wendy J. Deichman Edwards "Forging an Ideology for American Missions: Josiah Strong and Manifest Destiny," in *North American Foreign Missions, 1810–1914*, William R. Shenk, ed. (Grand Rapids, MI: Eerdmans Publishing, 2004), 178.
29 Walter A. McDougall, *The Tragedy of U.S. Foreign Policy: How America's Civil Religion Betrayed the National Interest* (New Haven: Yale University Press, 2016), 270.
30 Thompson and Wellman, p. 21.
31 Truman State University houses the collected papers of Harry Laughlin. For information on the impact of his Model Eugenical Sterilization Law, see "Laughlin's Model Law" at the Harry Laughlin and Eugenics archive website. Online: http://historyofeugenics.truman.edu/altering-lives/sterilization/model-law/, accessed February 7, 2018.
32 The logic of the law rests upon the simple determination of a dominant/recessive gene pattern in which the "socially inadequate" characteristics are recessive and the desirable racial and class characteristics are dominant. The scientific flaw – apart from the blatant racism of the concept – is the theory that such "socially inadequate" characteristics are the result of a singular genetic factor. The text of the model law can be found at Harry Laughlin, *Eugenical Sterilization in the United States* (Chicago: Psychopathic Laboratory of the Municipal Court, 1922), 446–451.
33 Melinda J. Wilde and Sabrina Danielson, "Fewer and Better Children: Race, Class, Religion, and Birth Control Reform in America," in *American Journal of Sociology* 119, no. 6 (2014): 1711.
34 Ibid., p. 1721.
35 Those bodies were the Reformed Church in the United States, Methodist Episcopal Church South, Conservative Judaism, Reformed Church in America, United Lutheran Church in America, Disciples of Christ, African Methodist Episcopal Zion Church, Churches of Christ, and the National Baptists Churches USA. See Wilde and Danielson, p. 1712.
36 Megan Vaughan, *Curing Their Ills: Colonial Power and African Illness* (Malden, MA: Polity Press, 2007), 141.
37 Ibid., p. 140.
38 See Vaughan, chapter six, "*Syphilis and Sexuality: The Limits of Colonial Power*," especially pp. 140–142.
39 J.H. Kellogg, "Finis," in *The Medical Missionary* 23, no. 12 (1914): 354. Online: https://babel.hathitrust.org/cgi/pt?id=mdp.39015071512134, accessed February 7, 2018.
40 John Harvey Kellogg, "The Race Betterment Foundation," in *Good Health: The Oldest Health Magazine in America* 49, no. 12 (1914), 609–610, Online: https://babel.hathitrust.org/cgi/pt?id=uiuo.ark:/13960/t18k9x456, accessed February 7, 2018. The Reverend Newell Dwight Hillis, Pastor of Plymouth Church, Brooklyn who advocated for the sterilization of 10,000,000 German soldiers, sat on the Advisory Board of the foundation. See p. 610.

41 Willard H. Smith, "William Jennings Bryan and the Social Gospel," in *The Journal of American History* 53, no. 1 (1966): 60.
42 Smith, pp. 42–43.
43 Matthew A. Tontonoz, "The Scopes Trial Revisited: Social Darwinism versus Social Gospel," in *Science as Culture* 17, no 2 (2008): 121–143.
44 Such a perspective was woven into the plot of the movie Inherit the Wind, which tells the story of the Scopes Monkey Trial. The movie, which starred Spencer Tracy and Gene Kelly, was adapted from the successful Broadway play. The premiere was held in a drive-in theatre just outside of Dayton. In a 2005 story on the trial which was aired on National Public Radio, reporter Noah Adams interviewed Dayton resident Eloise Reed, who had been 12 years old at the time of the trial:

> ADAMS: In 1960, "Inherit the Wind" became a movie, a starring role for Spencer Tracy. The premiere was in Dayton at the drive-in outside of town. And afterwards at a reception, Eloise Reed told the director, Stanley Kramer, she thought the movie was terrible, and so did her friends.
>
> Ms. REED: It belittled our town. They showed all of the ugliness that they could get into it to make it look like a little bitty borough or something, you know. It was the way they portrayed us because we didn't believe in the theory, or maybe not that, but we didn't want it taught. We didn't care. We didn't give a hoot whether they taught it in the school or not. That's all right. They couldn't make the people 'round here believe it.

See Noah Adams, *Timeline: Remembering the Scopes Monkey Trial, on All Things Considered* (radio news show, Washington, DC, 5 July 2005). The audio recording of the piece can be found at www.npr.org/2005/07/05/4723956/timeline-remembering-the-scopes-monkey-trial and the transcript at www.npr.org/templates/transcript/transcript.php?storyId=4723956, accessed February 10, 2018.
45 Matthew Tontonoz, "The Scopes Monkey Trial Revisited: Social Darwinism Versus Social Gospel," in *Science as Culture* 17, no. 2 (2008): 121–143. Bryan never made the closing argument at the trial. Darrow was afraid that he would be bested by Bryan's rhetorical skills and so he did not offer a closing argument. As a result, Bryan was not permitted to offer one either. The text of his argument was published in the *New York Times* on July 29, 1925 following Bryan's unexpected death.
46 Andrew Nolan, "Making Modern Men: The Scopes Trial, Masculinity and Modern Progress in the 1920s United States," in *Gender and History* 19, no. 1 (2007): 129.
47 Fishburn, pp. 220–225.
48 Ron Chernow, *Titan: The Life of John D. Rockefeller, Sr.* (New York: Vintage, 1998), 52–53.
49 Ibid., p. 189.
50 Ibid.
51 Ida M. Tarbell, "John D. Rockefeller: A Character Study," in *McClures* 25, no. 3 (1905): 233.
52 John Steele Gordon, "John D. Rockefeller Sr." Philanthropy Roundtable: Strengthening our Free Society, accessed February 16, 2018. www.philanthropyroundtable.org/almanac/hall_of_fame/john_d._rockefeller_sr
53 Robert Moats Miller, "Harry Emerson Fosdick and John D. Rockefeller, Jr.: The Origins of an Enduring Association," in *Foundations: A Baptist Journal of History and Theology* 21, no. 4 (1978): 294.
54 All references to Rockefeller's donations to colleges and universities unless otherwise noted in a separate endnote come from Kenneth W. Rose, "John D. Rockefeller, the American Baptist Education Society, and the Growth of Baptist Higher Education in the West" (presentation, Great Lakes American Studies Association, Cleveland, OH, October 13, 1990). Online: http://rockarch.org/publications/resrep/rose1.pdf.
55 This earlier school was also known as the University of Chicago or Chicago University. The school operated between 1856 and 1886 but was never on sound financial footing. When a new university was chartered in 1890, the trustees of the original institution legally changed the name of the school to the Old University of Chicago.
56 Vada L. Avery, *Philanthropy in Black Higher Education: A Fateful Hour Creating the Atlanta University System* (New York: Palgrave Macmillan, 2013), 40.

57 Other schools in the Atlanta University Center include Clark-Atlanta University, the Morehouse School of Medicine, Morris Brown College, and the Interdenominational Theological Center.
58 Anthony Gokianluy, "Storied beginnings and strong foundations," The Chicago Maroon, last modified February 14, 2012, www.chicagomaroon.com/2012/02/14/storied-beginnings-and-strong-foundations/
59 For example, in 1892, the Society listed "sundry contributions of $684 and a single contribution from Rockefeller for $165,000. See Rose, p. 9.
60 Of those schools, 18 are still open today. They are Baylor University, Bucknell University, California College (today, the American Baptist Seminary of the West), Carson-Newman College, the University of Chicago, Colby College, Franklin College, Furman University, William Jewell College, Kalamazoo College, Keystone Academy (today, Keystone College), Mercer University, Mississippi College, Ottawa University, Southwestern Baptist University (today Union University), Spelman Seminary (today, Spelman College), Stetson University, and Williamsburg Institute (today, University of the Cumberlands). For a complete list of the schools, see Rose, endnote 2.
61 "Rockefeller Gifts Total $530,853,632," *The New York Times* (New York, NY), May 24, 1937, p. 1, 10. The *New York Times* devoted the upper right columns of its front page to Rockefeller's death in three different stories. That day's edition also included three full pages of coverage of Rockefeller's life and death on pp. 8–10.
62 Miller (1978), p. 302.
63 Mark Tooley, "'Fundamentalism' Invades Manhattan," *American Spectator*, August 31, 2009, Online: https://spectator.org/40992_fundamentalism-invades-manhattan/, accessed March 17, 2018.
64 Robert Moats Miller, *Harry Emerson Fosdick: Preacher, Pastor, Prophet* (New York: Oxford University Press, 1985), viii.
65 Dana L. Robert, "The First Globalization: The Internationalization of the Protestant Missionary Movement Between the World Wars," in *International Bulletin of Mission Research* 26, no. 2 (2002): 53.
66 Robert Moats Miller, "John D. Rockefeller Jr.: An Exchange," in *New York Review of Books* 51, no. 12 (2004), www.nybooks.com/articles/2004/07/15/john-d-rockefeller-jr-an-exchange/
67 www.itc.edu/about/history/
68 Online: http://fteleaders.org/about/history
69 Walter R. Lambuth, *Medical Missions: The Two-fold Task* (New York: Student Volunteer Movement for Foreign Missions, 1920), 185–186.
70 Randall M. Packard, *A History of Global Health: Interventions into the Lives of Other People* (Baltimore: Johns Hopkins University Press, 2016), 32.
71 Ibid., p. 54.
72 "Our History," The Rockefeller Foundation, accessed February 17, 2018. www.rockefellerfoundation.org/about-us/our-history/
73 Ibid., p. 43. Packard does not cite the schools but the Foundation's website notes that it spent over $25 million between 1921 and 1941 to establish schools of public health in "Prague, Warsaw, London, Toronto, Copenhagen, Budapest, Oslo, Belgrade, Zagreb, Madrid, Cluj (Romania), Ankara, Sofia, Rome, Tokyo, Athens, Bucharest, Stockholm, Calcutta, Manila, and São Paulo. The total contribution to schools of public health amounts to $357 million in current dollars." See "Our History."
74 Marianne Jehle-Wildberger, *Adolph Keller: Ecumenist, World Citizen, Philanthropist* (Eugene, OR: Cascade Books, 2013), 236.
75 Charlene Mires, *Capital of the World: The Race to Host the United Nations* (New York: New York University Press, 2013), 213–214.
76 Thomas Robbins, *In Gods We Trust: New Patterns of Religious Pluralism in America* (New York: Routledge, 2017), 169.
77 Inderjeet Paramar, *Foundations of the American Century: The Ford, Carnegie, & Rockefeller Foundations in the Rise of American Power* (New York: Columbia University Press, 2012). See chapter four, "Promoting Americanism, Combating Anti-Americanism, and Developing a Cold War American Studies Network."
78 Claude C. Erb, "Prelude to Point Four: The Institute of Inter-American Affairs," in *Diplomatic History* 9, no. 3 (1985): 253.

79 Winged Scourge, directed by Bill Justice and Bill Roberts (Walt Disney Picture, 1943), Online: https://archive.org/details/gov.archives.arc.47063, accessed February 18, 2018.
80 Defense Against Invasion, directed by Jack King (Walt Disney Pictures, 1943), Online: https://archive.org/details/DefenseAgainstInvasion, accessed February 18, 2018.
81 Quoted in Erb, pp. 265–266.
82 Ibid., pp. 266–267.
83 Harry S. Truman, *Inaugural Address* (speech, Washington, DC, January 19, 1949), The American Presidency Project, www.presidency.ucsb.edu/ws/index.php?pid=13282&st=inaugural&st1=, accessed February 18, 2018.

References

Adams, Noah. "Timeline: Remembering the Scopes Monkey Trial." All Things Considered. Radio news show, Washington, DC, 5 July 2005. www.npr.org/2005/07/05/4723956/timeline-remembering-the-scopes-monkey-trial. Accessed February 10, 2018.

Bateman, Bradley W. "Clearing the Ground: The Decline of the Social Gospel and the Rise of Neoclassicism in American Economics." *History of Political Economy* 30, supplemental volume (1998): 29–52.

Behr, Edward. *Prohibition: Fifteen Years that Changed America*. New York: Arcade Publishing, 1996.

Bennett, John Coleman. "After Liberalism—What?" *Christian Century* 50 (8 November 1933): 1403–1406.

Berger, Peter. *The Sacred Canopy: Elements of a Sociological Theory of Religion*. Garden City, NY: Doubleday, 1967.

Coe, George Albert. *The Psychology of Religion*. Chicago: University of Chicago Press, 1916.

Deichman Edwards, Wendy J. "Forging an Ideology for American Missions: Josiah Strong and Manifest Destiny," *North American Foreign Missions, 1810–1914*, ed. William R. Shenk, 163–191. Grand Rapids, MI: Eerdmans Publishing, 2004.

Earp, Edwin. *The Social Engineer*. New York: Eaton and Mains, 1911.

Fishburn, Janet F. "The Social Gospel as Missionary Ideology." *North American Foreign Missions, 1810–1914*, ed. William R. Shenk, 218–242. Grand Rapids, MI: Eerdmans Publishing, 2004.

Fiske, Charles. *The Confessions of a Puzzled Parson*. New York: Charles Scribner, 1928.

Foucault, Michel. "Lecture of 19 February 1975." in *Abnormal: Lectures at the College de France 1974–1975*. New York: Picador, 1999.

Gorgas, William. "Tropical Sanitation in Its Relation to General Sanitation." *The Journal of the American Medical Association* 65, no. 26 (1915): 2207–2209.

Griscom, John. *The Sanitary Condition of the Laboring Poor of New York*. New York: Harper & Brothers, 1845.

Handy, Robert T. "The American Religious Depression, 1925–1935." *Church History* 29, no. 1 (1960): 3–16.

Harding, S. "American Protestant Moralism and the Secular Imagination: From Temperance to the Moral Majority." *Social Research* 76, 4 (Winter 2009): 1277–1306.

Hocking, William. *Re-Thinking Missions: A Laymen's Inquiry After One Hundred Years*. New York: Harper & Brothers, 1932.

Kellogg, John Harvey. "The Race Betterment Foundation." *Good Health: The Oldest Health Magazine in America* 49, no. 12 (1914), 609–610. https://babel.hathitrust.org/cgi/pt?id=uiuo.ark:/13960/t18k9x456. Accessed February 7, 2018.

Kellogg, John Harvey. "Finis." *The Medical Missionary* 23, no. 12 (1914): 354. https://babel.hathitrust.org/cgi/pt?id=mdp.39015071512134. Accessed February 7, 2018.

King, William McGuire. "The Emergence of Social Gospel Radicalism: The Methodist Case." *Church History* 50, no. 4 (Dec., 1981): 436–449.

Lambuth, Walter R. *Medical Missions: The Two-fold Task*. New York: Student Volunteer Movement for Foreign Missions, 1920.

Laughlin, Harry. *Eugenical Sterilization in the United States*. Chicago: Psychopathic Laboratory of the Municipal Court, 1922.

Levine, Harry Gene. "The Committee of Fifty and the Origins of Alcohol Control." *Journal of Drug Issues* 13, no. 1 (1983): 95–116.

Luccock, Halford. "The Resurrection of Jesus Taking Place Today." *Through the of Youth*, eds. Halford Luccock and William Reid, 165–176. New York: Abingdon, 1924.

McDougall, Walter. *Promised Land: Crusader State: The American Encounter with the World Since 1776*. New York: Houghton Mifflin, 1997.

McDougall, Walter A. *The Tragedy of U.S. Foreign Policy: How America's Civil Religion Betrayed the National Interest*. New Haven: Yale University Press, 2016.

Miller, Robert Moats. The Church Must Go Beyond Modernism: A Faith That Could Not Be Shaken. In *Harry Emerson Fosdick: Preacher, Pastor, Prophet*, 389–417. New York: Oxford, 1985.

Nolan, Andrew. "Making Modern Men: The Scopes Trial, Masculinity and Modern Progress in the 1920s United States." *Gender and History* 19, no. 1 (2007): 122–142.

Packard, Randall M. *A History of Global Health: Interventions into the Lives of Other People*. Baltimore: Johns Hopkins University Press, 2016.

Peabody, Francis. "Introduction." In *The Liquor Problem: A Summary of Investigations Conducted by The Committee of Fifty*. New York: Houghton, Mifflin, and Company, 1905.

Pearson, Ralph L. "Internationalizing the Social Gospel: The Federal Council of Churches and European Protestantism, 1914–1925." *Historical Magazine of the Protestant Episcopal Church* 52, no. 3 (1983): 275–292.

Rorabaugh, W. J. *The Alcoholic Republic: An American Tradition*. New York: Oxford University Press.

Smith, Willard H. "William Jennings Bryan and the Social Gospel." *The Journal of American History* 53, no. 1 (1966): 41–60.

Thompson, S. R. and James K. Wellman. "The Social Gospel Legacy in U.S. Foreign Policy." *Interdisciplinary Journal of Research on Religion* 7, article 6 (2011): 1–41.

Tittle, Ernest Fremont. *What Must the Church Do to be Saved? And Other Discussions*. New York: Abingdon, 1921.

Tontonoz, Matthew A. "The Scopes Trial Revisited: Social Darwinism Versus Social Gospel." *Science as Culture* 17, no. 2 (2008): 121–143.

Tooley, Mark. "'Fundamentalism' Invades Manhattan." American Spectator, August 31, 2009. https://spectator.org/40992_fundamentalism-invades-manhattan/. Accessed March 17, 2018.

Vaughan, Megan. *Curing Their Ills: Colonial Power and African Illness*. Malden, MA: Polity Press, 2007.

Webb, Holland. "Temperance Movements and Prohibition." *International Social Science Review* 74, no. 1/2 (1999): 61–69.

Welch, Herbert. "The Church and Social Service." *Methodist Review* 24, no. 5 (1908): 707–715.

Wilde, Sabrina J. and Sabrina Danielson. "Fewer and Better Children: Race, Class, Religion, and Birth Control Reform in America." *American Journal of Sociology* 119, no. 6 (2014): 1710–1760.

Wilson, Woodrow. "Address to a Joint Session of Congress on the Conditions for Peace." Speech, Washington, DC, January 8, 1918. The American Presidency Project, www.presidency.ucsb.edu/ws/index.php?pid=65405&st=&st1=. Accessed February 5, 2018.

Wilson, Woodrow. "Address Delivered to the First Annual Assemblage of the League to Enforce Peace: 'American Principles.'" Speech, Washington, DC, May 27, 1916. The American Presidency Project, www.presidency.ucsb.edu/ws/?pid=65391. Accessed February 4, 2108.

Worboys, Michael. "The Colonial World as Mission and Mandate: Leprosy and Empire, 1900–1940." *Osiris* 15 (2000): 207–218.

4 In-depth Christianization

Evangelists, engineers, and reconstructionists

Theological crises roil the Social Gospel

As the world braced for another global war in the closing days of the 1930s, American Protestantism was trying to come to terms with the centrifugal forces that were splintering the unity displayed less than two decades earlier. Liberal Protestants in the vanguard of the Social Gospel movement were bewildered and defeated: "today we are passing through a period of religious depression not less severe than the concomitant moral and economic depression."[1]

This religious depression was clearly felt in foreign missions, which had been in decline by most measures for a decade. At the 1926 meeting of the Foreign Missions Conference of North America, missionary leaders bemoaned the apathy of local churches and church historian Robert Handy noted that offerings to missions boards had been declining throughout the 1920s, well before the stock market crash of 1929, noting that per capita annual giving had dropped by 39% in the decade. The decline was not only monetary. In 1920, 2,700 Protestant young adults volunteered for foreign missions service; in 1928, that number was only 252.[2] Under these falling fortunes, mainline Protestants decided to re-think missions.

For two years, from 1930–1932, a commission comprised of representatives from seven Protestant denominations—Baptists, Congregationalists, Dutch Reformed, Episcopalian, Methodist Episcopal, Presbyterian, and United Presbyterian—carried out an extensive assessment of Protestant foreign missions. In 1932, the commission published their findings in *Re-Thinking Missions: A Laymen's Inquiry After One Hundred Years*. The foreword to the published report alludes to the shifting fortunes of foreign missions over the 1920s:

> In an era during which channels for giving to beneficent purposes have multiplied almost beyond reckoning, this enterprise has until very recent years not only held its own, but shown remarkable growth. Relying as it has upon the steadfastness of certain attitudes of mind and will, its very magnitude has rendered it vulnerable to any change which might affect those attitudes.

> In the last few years there have been signs of such change. The old fervor appears to have been succeeded in some quarters by questionings if not by indifference. Subscriptions have been falling off. Problems of the utmost gravity face mission boards in nearly all fields. There is a growing conviction that the mission enterprise is at a fork in the road, and that momentous decisions are called for.[3]

The members of the commission explicitly name the technological and scientific advances of the time as a "change affecting mission" to bring about a more enlightened Christian religion:

> Western Christianity has in the main shifted its stress from the negative to the affirmative side of its message; it is less a religion of fear and more a religion of beneficence. It has passed through and beyond the stage of bitter conflict with the scientific consciousness of the race over details of the mode of creation, the age of the earth, the descent of man, miracle and law, to the stage of maturity in which a free religion and a free science become inseparable and complementary elements in a complete world-view.[4]

The report reflects on a hundred years of American Protestant foreign mission activities. Over those years, there had been an ongoing debate in the mission enterprise: was the medical missionary's primary purpose evangelism with medical care an instrument in support of that primary purpose or could medical care be offered as a legitimate activity of the missionary on its own? The commission argued "that the relief of suffering may be of itself a genuine interpretation of the Christian spirit . . . All that is an essential part of medical mission work will eventually be regarded as an end in itself, as one of the ways of liberating and enlarging life. And when this work is done 'in the name of a disciple,' the hospital, quite without any pressure of preaching and prayer in the wards, may be as truly a place where human and divine love are revealed as is the most religious sanctuary."[5] In the final conclusions of the report, the commission members claim that

> It is our conviction that medical missions represent, in themselves, the essentials of the Christian enterprise. The use of medical skill for ulterior ends has been rightly challenged, in our judgment . . . The use of medical or other professional service as a direct means of making converts, or public services in wards and dispensaries from which patients cannot escape, is subtly coercive, and improper.[6]

The representatives of seven different Protestant denominations who comprised the Commission responded to the technological and social changes facing the American religious scene by articulating a Protestantism aligned with a scientific worldview. The members in the pews did not agree. The *Laymen's Inquiry* was rejected by the membership of all seven denominations. The primary purpose of missions remained a subject of sharp debate. But the issues, in fact, were far more encompassing than missions alone—the primary focus of Christianity in America was now a subject of sharp debate among Protestants who had just a decade before been largely unified in their commitment to a social reform agenda, despite theological and cultural differences. In short, Protestants no longer agreed upon the processes by which the transfer of the empire of the world would be accomplished.

In 1927, the influential neo-Orthodox theologian Reinhold Niebuhr remarked that "a psychology of defeat, of which both fundamentalism and modernism are symptoms, has gripped the forces of religion." By 1928, the Episcopal Bishop of Central New York, Charles Fiske, was convinced "of a sad disintegration of American Protestantism."[7] He further claimed that

> America has become almost hopelessly enamoured of a religion that is little more than a sanctified commercialism; it is hard in this day and this land to differentiate between religious aspiration and business prosperity. Our conception of God is that he is a sort of Magnified Rotarian. Sometimes, indeed, one wonders whether the social movement and the uplift in general have not become, among Protestants, a substitute for devotion; worse than that, a substitute for real religion. Efficiency has become the greatest of Christian virtues. I hope I may be forgiven a note of exaggeration that is necessary to make my meaning clear when I say that Protestantism, in America, seems to be degenerating into a sort of cult, which cannot distinguish between what is offered to God and what is accomplished for the glory of America and the furtherance of business enterprise.[8]

Clearly, theological liberalism was in crisis. In a 1933 essay entitled *After Liberalism—What?*, theologian John Coleman Bennett declared:

> The most important fact about contemporary American theology is the disintegration of liberalism. Disintegration may seem too strong a word, but I am using it quite literally. It means that as a structure with a high degree of unity, theological liberalism is coming to pieces. The liberal preacher has had a coherent pattern of theological assumptions in the background of his message. He has often had the kind of self-confidence which goes with the preaching of an orthodoxy, for liberalism has been a new orthodoxy in many circles. It is that coherent pattern of assumptions, that self-confidence, which are going. Now many of us are left with a feeling of theological homelessness.[9]

Two years later, in 1935, preaching from Riverside Church in Manhattan, the High Temple of the Social Gospel, Harry Emerson Fosdick proclaimed that "The Church Must Go Beyond Modernism." He exclaimed,

> And in that new enterprise the watchword will be not, accommodate yourself to the prevailing culture! but, stand out from it and challenge it! For this inescapable fact, which again and again in Christian history has called modernism to its senses, we face: we cannot harmonize Christ himself with modern culture. What Christ does to modern culture is to challenge it.[10]

There was no talk about Christianizing the culture, but of challenging it, offering a prophetic corrective.

By some accounts, the social gospel declined sharply from this point forward before its eventual demise:

> the forces that swept the Social Gospel off the historical stage were themselves a part of the increasing secularization of American life and of a significantly altered vision within the Protestant community after the Second World War. Thus, from our perspective today, we cannot easily see what was important then; what was obvious has become nearly invisible.[11]

According to these accounts, mainline Protestantism fractured into a dizzying array of internally-focused movements and explicitly religious rhetoric melted away from the public discourse. America entered into an era of secularism and the commitment to social reform was transferred to non-religious (or privately religious) progressives who would never conceive of talking about the "Christianization of the social order."

That is not my argument, however. While acknowledging the crises besetting American Protestantism in these years, I will develop the claim not that Protestant visions of a Christianized society were abandoned but that they were transformed by being secularized and internationalized. There was, in short, an in-depth Christianization of the culture.

An "in-depth Christianization" of the culture

As a way to introduce this idea of an in-depth Christianization, I want to briefly recount an incident involving the French cultural historian, Michel Foucault. Foucault developed critical perspectives regarding power, medicine, and politics that challenge the field of global health and development. The incident I want to recount now, however, involves religion. In 1975, Foucault picked up a hitchhiker named Thierry Voeltzel. Voeltzel audio-taped their conversations. And that is what they were—conversations. They were informal in tone and the flows of topics occurred naturally as the conversation progressed. And so, while the transcript of the recording should not be read in the same way as one of Foucault's formal lectures, papers, or books, it does provide insight into his thinking as he was considering ideas in the moment. One of the topics explored was the nature of the church in France in 1975:

FOUCAULT: . . . I think the church is wonderful . . . Historically what exists is the church. Faith, what is that? Religion is a political force . . . It is a superb instrument of power for itself.

VOELTZEL: Oh yes, it's superb! I've seen what happens in church schools, this continual hypocrisy, those daily lies, this malice that you find in most people of the church. It is detestable, it is something I hate. . . . In any case I don't believe there are many people who take an interest in all that.

FOUCAULT: No, no doubtless not. There is only me left.[12]

Why would a French cultural historian who was an atheist and one of the architects of the postmodern turn in contemporary thought express an interest in religion and communicate his appreciation for the church as an instrument of power? And how could he profess such interest in 1975, when the academic study of religion was in thrall to the secularization thesis, or the idea that religion was inevitably withering away under the processes of secularization? Sociologist Peter Berger, one of the most influential scholars to articulate the secularization thesis (and one who later changed his mind and now claims that the thesis was incorrect), described the eclipse of religion in the face of secularization in his 1967 book *The Sacred Canopy:*

> One of the most obvious ways in which secularization has affected the man in the street is as a "crisis of credibility" in religion. Put differently, secularization has resulted in a widespread collapse of the plausibility of traditional religious definitions of reality. This manifestation of secularization on the level of consciousness has its correlate on the social-structural level. Subjectively, the man in the street tends to be uncertain about religious matters. Objectively, the man in the street is confronted with a wide variety of religious and other reality-defining agencies that compete for his allegiance or at least attention, and none of which is in a position to coerce him into allegiance. In other words, the phenomenon called "pluralism" is a social-structural correlate of the secularization of consciousness.[13]

Given the context of the mid 1970s and the general assumptions in many intellectual circles regarding religion during that period, Foucault's interest in religion is surprising. What is striking, however, is his claim—a claim that flew in the face of most academic assumptions about religion at the time—that religion was not going way but that it had insinuated itself into the deep structures and practices of Western societies:

> What I would like to consider now . . . is what took place in the sixteenth century, that is to say, in a period that is not characterized by the beginning of de-Christianization, but rather, as a number of historians have shown, by a phase of in-depth Christianization. The period that stretches from the Reformation to the witch-hunts, passing through the Council of Trent, is one in which the modern states begin to take shape while Christian structures tighten their grip on individual existence . . . All, or almost all, of an individual's life, thought, and action must pass through this filter of confession.[14]

Foucault explored this idea of an "in-depth Christianization" in the context of the social mechanisms that disciplined and normalized human beings in the seventeenth and eighteenth centuries as the modern democratic state was emerging out of European monarchies; he was not so interested in the progressive era of American history. And so, while he focuses for the most part of different historical eras in his own analyses, his claim that religion may not die as religious piety wanes in a society but "go deep" in the secular institutions of that society informs the idea that the Social Gospel did not so much wither away but disperse itself through other social systems outside of American Protestantism. In short, we will trace the ways in which American Protestant ideas and commitments informed both the emerging global health and development agenda not through religious institutions but as a broader social force.

Three new actors on the stage: the evangelist, the engineer, and the reconstructionist

Religious historian William McGuire King provides a useful conceptual model to help us trace this in-depth Christianization of the Social Gospel. In the early 1980s, King argued in an article on the history of the dissolution of the Social Gospel movement that three different actors emerged in the movement's formal breakdown: the evangelist, the engineer, and the reconstructionist.

King argued that the social gospel movement had been moderate by the standards of the Progressive era, seeking to establish a Christian order through reforming the existing structures rather than tearing those structures down so new ones could emerge. Wary of both unabashed capitalism and unchecked socialism, most leaders in the movement at this time believed that the strengths of each could check the weaknesses of the other. Some Social Gospel leaders, however, were far more critical of capitalism and enthused with socialism, seeing it "as the political organization most nearly approximating a political expression of Christian ethics for our day."[15] Eventually, differences in theology and politics, exacerbated by the social issues and movements described above, led to three different strands in Social Gospel Protestantism from the 1930s onward. One strand continued along as before, articulating Social Gospels ideals for a new context (social evangelists); one opted for employing social scientific research to help establish an ideal society that reflected the vision of a Christianized social order (social engineers); and one was convinced that fundamental problems existed with the structures that had created American society and those structures need to be dismantled and re-established (social reconstructionists).

For the first group, the social evangelists, the reforms dreamed of in the Social Gospel required reshaping social attitudes to establish a social norm of cooperation that would eventually establish altruism as an element of the nation's social fabric. Social evangelists were committed to a Christian, social utopia

> built by a church "whose business is not to keep itself pure and separate but to diffuse itself and leaven the whole lump of life. The mission of the church, in short, is to reorganize society on a Christian basis; to bring from God out of heaven the new Jerusalem by changing earth's cities into cities of God, with clean streets, pure water, no tears, no crime, no oppression; cities in which the church itself is lost sight of not because religion fails but because religion succeeds and turns the whole community into the habitation of God and of the Lamb . . . The Church of Jesus Christ can render its best service, not by devising economic schemes, or by proposing schedules of wages (for the church is not an economist), but, rather, by shaming low ideals, by overcoming greed, by opposing that lack of consideration between man and man which lies at the root of the trouble.[16]

Those in King's second strand, the social engineers, believed that the problem wasn't simply shifting individual attitudes so that the citizens would live out a moralized altruism already embedded but nascent in the nation's institutions. For these social engineers, the process of industrialization itself had created problems that earlier generations had not had to navigate.[17] The solution: experts in the newly developing social sciences could fashion responses through social service to get rid of social conflict and allow the earlier moral foundations to re-emerge. In his book *The Social Engineer*, the sociologist of religion Edwin Earp put it this way:

> All human life today is being socialized in consciousness and activity. In considering its ethical phase it should be understood at the outset that that modern movement for social service does not differ from other religious movements for moral reform so much in aim as in method or points of emphasis. It is a movement that involves organization of individuals, cooperation and federation of groups in mass-effort for the accomplishment of social tasks. It recognizes that the powers of evil today are socially organized, and therefore the

> salvation of society involves social methods and machinery in order to overthrow the organized powers of evil. . . .
>
> Social service is an intelligent, organized effort to eliminate the causes of social disorder through a readjustment of our economic and industrial system by wise statesmanship through social control, so that the profits of social production may be more equitably distributed to all classes of society.[18]

For those in the third strand, the social reconstructionists, the evangelists had underestimated the power of social institutions by focusing on individual morality. Further, the engineers had overestimated the capacity of social service to solve the misuse of that social power in the form of structural problems. This rendered the efforts of the Social Gospel ineffectual. For the reconstructionists, there had to be both a vision of social cooperation and a realistic appraisal regarding the challenges in achieving it. Reform was not a one-time phase that would usher in a better society; it was ongoing and required constant diligence. Instead, "Christianity demanded nothing less than a continuing 'revaluation of values and a reconstruction of life's enterprises.'"[19] For the social reconstructionists, absolute and complete social justice was not possible because society would never transcend the need for criticism, deliberation, and adjustment. This did not mean that we should not strive for justice but it did require an honest assessment of our own implications in unjust social practices and systems.[20]

Up to World War I, the social reconstructionists stayed in the Social Gospel movement in hopes that their calls for critique would gain ground. Eventually, however, their strong critique of capitalism, especially the union-busting actions of John Rockefeller, Jr. who was a primary financer of Protestant organizations that were the source of Social Gospel ideas and programs,[21] eventually led to breaches that could not be repaired. With the fault lines exposed, social reconstructionists now believed that cultural critique had become an ethical imperative. They embraced radicalism, not as an epithet but as a rallying cry. "'Certainly we are radicals!' exclaimed the *Social Service Bulletin*. 'Doesn't the word by its very derivation mean to go the roots of things?'"[22] Methodist bishop Francis McConnell spoke of "the salt of radical protest" (referencing the gospel quote of being the salt of the earth) and his peers developed the theme. Ernest Tittle, in *What Must the Church Do to be Saved*, declared that "the war has forced us to look beneath the appearance of things for it has blown away the veneer and laid bare the realities of our Western civilization."[23] In a similar vein, Halford Luccock claimed that

> the immediate danger is that the church itself will capitulate to modern business culture, that perfect peace will be the only anthem we will sing in regard to the industrial situation. In contrast to the peaceable Jesus of Christian capitalism the Jesus of radical Christianity is going into our complex life

> today—into the steel mill, into the sweatshop, into the coal mine, into the slum, into the cotton mill—and is demanding: Let my people go.[24]

To understand the impact of three movements—social evangelist, social engineer, and social reconstructionist—on the fields of global health and development from the 1930s into the present, we'll need to trace each one separately.

Evangelists

According to King's description, the Social Gospel evangelists dreamed of a global society in which the church was no longer separate but diffused throughout the social order to create a utopia free from want and illness and characterized by harmony and peace. Such social evangelists during the Inter-War period and in the first few years after the Second World War could easily be seen in Protestant efforts at international cooperation—efforts which would be key to the religious body known as the World Council of Churches and the global social-political body known as the United Nations.

To understand the ways in which Social Gospel principles were taken up by global institutions such as these in the middle decades of the twentieth century, we first need to quickly understand how Social Gospel leaders understood global affairs in the prior three decades. At the 1925 Foreign Missions Convention, Episcopal Bishop Charles Brent reflected the opinions of most liberal Protestants—the United States needed to enter the League of Nations and support the International Court:

> Now I come to what, to me, is the great opportunity of Christians and the greatest opportunity of this nation of ours. What is the relation of nation to nation today throughout the world? What does international intercourse mean? I have just come from the League of Nations, where, by appointment of our own Government, I sat as a plenipotentiary in an International Conference for the creation of a treaty or the amendment, rather, of a treaty, dealing with an extremely intricate and difficult problem a moral question, a question that has to do with commerce, a question that has to do with health.
>
> [The League of Nations] is a glorious endeavor, and the world has never seen anything like it before, it is taking the Christian ideal, if you read the first words of the Covenant, and trying to put it into practical form on an extensive scale. Then there is the World Court. I speak of these things, my friends, because they are Christian in their aim and in their possibilities.
>
> I am of the mind that every citizen who believes that in a democracy he has a living share in the legislation of his country, should watch legislation and use that powerful influence which is his to register what he thinks in Christian

> terms by telegrams and letters to Congressmen and Senators on any question of moment. Do not think for one minute that these telegrams and letters are put into the waste paper basket with little or no notice. Far from it. They are scrutinized with care. If the citizens of our country would register their Christian judgment on public questions in this way, we would have a higher type of legislation, and we would not have some of the legislation that is enacted.[25]

Of course, the country did not join the League of Nations and there was strong opposition to the Court; nonetheless, the advocacy of most Protestant leaders had been strong and sustained. Throughout the course of the First World War, Social Gospel leaders were united in their anti-war advocacy, channeling their efforts through the Federal Council of Churches (FCC). As the war was drawing to a close, the FCC leadership met in December of 1918 to articulate strong support for establishing a League of Nations and for the United States to enter into it. In different resolutions, the Council endorsed the establishment of the League, committed member churches to support proposals for establishing the League, and set a National Day of Prayer for the League. The Council lobbied the U.S Congress hard to join the League but were unsuccessful in their efforts and U.S. never joined the League.

Following these failures, the FCC turned their efforts to strengthening partnerships with Protestant bodies in Europe. In 1921, the FCC held a conference on the Responsibility of the American Churches Toward European Protestantism, followed by the Interdenominational Church Congress for investigating the Situation of Protestantism in Europe in 1922; 37 Christian bodies from twenty European countries participated. As an outcome of these meetings, Protestant leaders from the United States and Europe created a "Central Bureau for European Protestantism" in Geneva. The Bureau's first task was coordination of relief efforts in war-torn Europe. Despite these efforts, the FCC's literature reflected a growing frustration at the nation's failure to help solve the postwar problems besetting Europe through the channels of the United States government. The groundwork for the World Council of Churches was being put into place though that body would not come into being for another 25 years.

The 1925 Conference on Life and Work in Stockholm represented a formal, organized effort among Protestant Christians from North America and Europe to build stronger ties; even this movement, however, was impacted by the war that still remained vivid in the minds of participants. German Protestant leaders felt that the global ecumenical movement was being articulated and promoted by those nations which held all the power in the postwar world and argued that their country's suffering under the terms of the Treaty of Versailles left them wary of any claims that equated any human institutions with God's divine will. German voices implied not only that calls for international, ecumenical cooperation should not be confused with faithfulness to the distinctive life of Christian faith, they also implied that the move toward internationalism among Protestants was being used as a political instrument by the nations who held all the power in the postwar world.[26] Despite these misgivings, support for internationalization grew in Stockholm and in the subsequent meeting of the Faith and Work movement in Oxford, England in 1937. The Faith and Work movement among Protestants would be an organizing principle for the World Council of Churches (WCC) in the late 1940s. As the WCC grew, it would help shape global health and development policy, especially in the area of the primary health-care movement, as we shall see.

For American Protestants, the emphasis on internationalization in the Life and Work movement helped galvanize support for multilateral partnerships among many nations over bilateral alliances between two. This political issue had been a key concern for some members of the U.S. Congress that led to their vote against the country joining the League of Nations. Nonetheless, despite America's absence from the League, the religious ideals of liberal American Protestantism shaped the body. Raymond Fosdick, the brother of the senior pastor of Riverside Church Harry Emerson Fosdick, served as the first Under Secretary of the League of Nations and Harry preached the sermon at the opening ceremony of the League in 1925. That sermon, (offered at the Cathedral in Geneva where John Calvin, a leader of the Reformed tradition in Protestantism had preached) was an astounding blend of theology, internationalism, pacifism, and support for the League of Nations and the International Court:

> The old appeals for war in the name of a good cause fall coldly now on the instructed ear and cease to carry conviction to thoughtful minds . . . A modern war to protect the weak—that is a grim jest. See how modern war protects the weak: 10,000,000 known dead soldiers; 3,000,000 presumed dead soldiers; 13,000,000 dead civilians; 20,000,000 wounded; 3,000,000 prisoners; 9,000,000 war orphans; 5,000,000 war widows; 10,000,000 refugees . . . The conviction grows clear in increasing multitudes of minds that modern war is no way to protect the weak.
>
> A World Court would protect the weak. A League of Nations would protect the weak. An international mind, backed by a Christian conscience, that would stop the race for armaments, provide cooperative substitutes for violence, forbid the nations to resort to force, and finally outlaw war altogether—that would protect the weak. . . .
>
> We cannot reconcile Jesus Christ and war—that is the essence of the matter. That is the challenge which today should stir the conscience of Christendom. War is the most colossal and ruinous social sin that afflicts mankind; it is utterly and irremediably unchristian; in its total method and effect it means everything that Jesus did not mean and it means nothing that He did mean; it is a more blatant denial of every Christian doctrine about God and man than all the theoretical atheists on earth ever could devise. . . .

> Here today, as an American, under this high and hospitable roof, I cannot speak for my government, but both as an American and as a Christian I do speak for millions of my fellow citizens in wishing your great work, in which we believe, for which we pray, our absence from which we painfully regret, the eminent success which it deserves. We work in many ways for the same end—a world organized for peace. Never was an end better worth working for. The alternative is the most appalling catastrophe mankind has ever faced. Like gravitation in the physical realm, the law of the Lord in the moral realm bends for no man and no nation: "All they that take the sword shall perish with the sword."[27]

American Protestant leaders such as Fosdick could not foresee the magnified horrors of the Second World War that would erupt in the coming decade; neither could they see the impact of their ideas on the United Nations, that international body that would come into being following that war. Even as the war raged in 1943, Protestant leaders remained firm in their support of the United States becoming part of a global governmental body. This time, politicians took note, in large part because of Roosevelt's popularity—a popularity never matched by Woodrow Wilson, whom the British Prime Minister David Lloyd George had described as someone who "believed in mankind but mistrusted all men."[28] Joseph Ball, a Republican Senator from Minnesota told a convention at the Episcopal Cathedral of St. John the Divine in New York that the drive to establish a world organization was "the greatest crusade since Jesus sent his twelve disciples to preach the brotherhood of man." Of course, not every member of Congress saw these efforts as directly ordained by God. Tom Connolly, a Democratic Senator from Texas and chair of the Senate Foreign Relations Committee, claimed, "God damn it, everybody's running around here like a fellow with a tick in his navel, howling about postwar resolutions." However, with polls showing that the three-quarters of the American people supported the nation's entry into some global body, the vote was decisive, and the Senate ended up supporting the nation's entry into the global body to be formed after that war by a vote of 85 to five.[29] Of course, no one knew exactly what that body would be at the time. Protestant leaders, however, played a decisive role in its establishment. Through secular systems, these leaders sincerely believed they were building a structure to transfer the empire of the world

In the war's aftermath a group of international Protestant leaders from the World Council of Churches-in-formation worked to build a global, ecumenical and political movement based on their understanding that a society reflecting Christian values required "optimal secular conditions." The Reverend John Nurser, a former Fellow at the Human Rights Centre at the University of Essex, England, argues that that by most measures these leaders were quite successful in these efforts when one examines their influence in the formation of the United Nations (UN).[30] In 1940, a commission on a just and durable peace was developed and chaired by John Foster

Dulles (later to be U.S. Secretary of State under President Eisenhower). The WCC-in-formation focused on the issue of human rights, exerting great influence on the Commission on Human Rights in the UN. Otto Frederick Nolde, a professor at Lutheran Theological Seminary in Philadelphia, played a key role in establishing the commission and in securing passage of the Universal Declaration of Human Rights.

Though the influence of this body is not widely remembered, John Foster Dulles claimed that "the character of the United Nations organization was very largely determined by the organized Christian forces which worked at San Francisco to complete what had been achieved at Bretton Woods."[31] Even after the horrors of the War, these religious leaders held firm to their earlier vision of a global community that could be structured in support of peace and shared economic resources. But they also believed this vision could only be achieved through a spiritual ethos that would unite the nations of the world. Nurser argued that the Universal Declaration of Human Rights "eventually became the creedal expression of that ethos."[32] They were, in short, evangelists more than engineers.

The active advocacy efforts of these leaders had far-reaching implications. First, their efforts led to the creation of the Churches Commission on International Affairs (CCIA), a body dually aligned with the World Council of Churches and the International Missionary Council, with O. Frederick Nolde as the first director. As a civil society body representing global Protestantism, the CCIA was granted consultancy status during the process for drafting the Charter of the United Nations; the body would maintain that status with the UN for another 21 years. Second, through the CCIA's official status, these leaders had a seat at the table during the process for proposing amendments to the United Nations Charter that was drafted at the San Francisco Conference in 1945. Their participation was instrumental in securing the inclusion of a Commission on Human Rights into the UN Charter and Nolde was a key leader in drafting in drafting the Universal Declaration of Human Rights; the wording of Article 18 on freedom of religious expression came from Nolde, who insisted that this issue be explicitly addressed in the Declaration.

The Declaration and Commission on Human Rights had been proposed as part of the UN charter during the amendments process but there was no guarantee that nations' representatives would support it. Many representatives wondered if the U.S. delegation would affirm either the Declaration or the Commission and the religious leaders wondered if their advocacy efforts would fail once again as they had in trying to convince the Congress to join the League of Nations a generation before. This time, however, the leaders found success. Although Protestant unity was no longer guaranteed and many Protestant leaders had a history of anti-Catholic and anti-Jewish animus, the American representatives on the CCIA mobilized the Federal Council of Churches, the American Jewish Committee, 12 separate Roman Catholic bishops, and the Baptist Joint Conference Committee on Public Relations. All of these bodies actively advocated for the Declaration and the Commission and the American delegates committed to support the Commission and the

Declaration in principle. It would take another three years to draft, but in 1948, the Universal Declaration of Human Rights was finalized in the United Nations and Nolde was involved in each step of the process. In the coming decades, both the UN agencies and the World Council of Churches would form a number of joint initiatives in the field of international health and development, most notably in the primary health care movement.

Engineers

The World Health Organization has shifted in its program priorities at various points in time to encourage more community engagement and collaborative processes. Nonetheless, since its founding the WHO's primary focus has been to employ the technical capacities and knowledge of experts to improve population health. Similarly, the United Nations Development Programme (UNDP) was founded in 1966 by the merger of two earlier UN programs which prioritized technical capacity and expertise: the Expanded Programme for Technical Assistance and the Special Fund (which provided mechanisms for financing economic development projects). And so, much like the WHO, the UNDP has focused on technical expertise as the foundation for development initiatives. Other UN agencies that address health and development have adopted similar models. Finally, the U.S. Centers for Disease Control and Prevention (CDC) lists eight core strengths in its 2015 Global Health Strategy:

- Providing Technical Expertise
- Implementing Evidence-Based Public Health Programs
- Developing Surveillance and Strategic Information Systems
- Translating Research into Public Health Policy and Practice
- Building Public Health Workforce Capacity
- Strengthening Laboratory Systems
- Improving Emergency Preparedness and Response Capabilities, and
- Conducting Monitoring and Evaluation Activities[33]

In short, global health and development programs for the last 70 years have been conceptualized, developed, operated, and managed by the group King named as engineers—a group committed to the "organized effort to eliminate the causes of social disorder through a readjustment of our economic and industrial system by wise statesmanship." Obviously, not all the technical experts who work in the fields of global health and development today would see themselves as the heirs of the Social Gospel; many would likely reject any connection between their work and any religious influence. But that is not the point of King's piece or the argument being advanced that the secularization of the Social Gospel resulted in an in-depth Christianization. On the contrary, the high level of alignment between the heirs of the Social Gospel within Protestantism who take on the engineer role and the broader priorities of global health and development on technical capacity formulated outside of any religious context demonstrate the ways in which the vision of the Social Gospel was carried forth in part by engineers working in these global health and development frameworks. Two global leaders in these organizations offer such a demonstration: William (Bill) Foege at the CDC and James Grant at UNICEF.

Bill Foege and smallpox eradication

Bill Foege is rightly credited as a key figure in the effort to remove smallpox from the face of the earth. Having been trained as a medical doctor and an epidemiology intelligence officer in the US Public Health Service, Foege served first in Nigeria and later in India on national smallpox programs before moving on to spearhead the CDC's global campaign, the first successful effort to eradicate a disease from the earth in the history of humankind. Having been awarded the Presidential Medal of Freedom for these efforts in 2012 by President Obama, Bill Foege is a public health legend.

He is also the son of a Lutheran pastor, the nephew of a medical missionary, and a medical missionary himself; medical missions took him to Liberia in the 1960s.[34] Foege embodied an approach to medical missions put forth in the *Rethinking Missions* that saw the provision of health care as a faithful response to Christian faith and not merely as a tool for proselytization. In his book recounting the smallpox eradication campaign, Foege wrote,

> It had always disturbed me that church groups did so much medical work in developing countries yet took so little responsibility for disease prevention. Mission boards rarely encouraged it, even though prevention is the most efficient use of limited resources. This of course made them little different from health care delivery systems in the United States. A June 1965 response I received from the Board of Foreign Missions of the United Lutheran Church of America was typical: "Our medical personnel are unable to do much in preventive medicine on a community scale. Understaffing and time limit what they can do in this area." The board had missed the point. One possible explanation for this stance is that medical work had become such a useful proselytizing tool. Clinics and hospitals attract people and can leave them feeling indebted after they have received help. I always felt that was wrong. Churches should be working because of what they believe, not because of what they are trying to get other people to believe.[35]

Bill Foege went on to serve as Director of the CDC under both Presidents Carter and Reagan and served as the Executive Director of the Carter Center alongside

President Carter. While there, he founded the Interfaith Health Program (IHP), an initiative to build partnerships between religious and public health leaders and experts to address the social and economic factors that contribute to health disparities. IHP is still active today as a program in the Rollins School of Public Health at Emory University;[36] Foege's legacy in public health and religion has been a catalyst for interdisciplinary research and practice at Emory, which has a university-wide program in the field called the Religion and Public Health Collaborative.

Bill Foege may have embodied many of the ideals of medical missions informed by the Social Gospel but he has built an exemplary career in the public health sciences, opting for the role of a social engineer over that of social evangelist. Foege's reliance on sound science and technical expertise is reflected in his career, which continues to this day. His knowledge and skill as a researcher and public health scientist became the focus of Foege's life, as Jim Yong Kim, the current President of the World Bank, stated in a piece he wrote on Bill Foege in 2007:

> Foege . . . may have started his life's work in a church, but his career has been defined by his belief in scientific solutions to the most difficult problems. His is a world of cause and effect: By understanding the science of the cause, he has proved, man can change the effect.[37]

In 1984, Foege left the CDC to become Director of the Task Force for Child Survival. At that point, global immunization coverage of children was stuck at approximately 20%, well short of the WHO's goal of immunizing 80% of the world's children by 1990.[38] Under the leadership of Bill Foege, the Social Gospel engineer, and with the technical capacity of the Task Force, immunization rates climbed to 80% over the next six years, meeting the WHO's goal. Foege worked closely with both the WHO and with UNICEF—the United Nation Children's Fund—on these efforts. In fact, UNICEF director James Grant called the global childhood immunization effort "the largest peacetime mobilization in the history of the earth."[39] Grant and Foege worked closely together on this effort; perhaps one of the reasons for their strong collaboration was their shared history in medical missions.

James Grant and UNICEF

Jim Grant served as Director of UNICEF from 1980 until his death in 1995. A lawyer by training, Grant had served in the U.S. State Department during John F. Kennedy's administration and as a regional administrator for US AID until he joined UNICEF. Grant's grandfather, James Skiffington Grant from New Brunswick, Canada, was appointed a medical missionary to China by the Baptist Foreign Missions Society. John Black Grant, son of James Skiffington and father of Jim, was born in China and returned to Canada and the United States for college, medical school, and the public health program at Johns Hopkins. After a few short stints on public health projects in the US, John returned to China with the Rockefeller Foundation where he served as professor in public health at Peking Union Medical College, the university founded by the Rockefeller Foundation drawing on the family's commitments to medical missions.

Jim Grant was born and raised in China, the third generation in his family to call the nation home. He returned to the United States for college, opting to pursue a career in law over medicine. Though Grant did not have a public health background, his family's generational commitments to public health practice influenced Grant's priorities at UNICEF. Under Grant's leadership and working closely with Bill Foege and the leadership of other global health organizations, UNICEF adopted the "GOBI approach" for pediatric health care, which focuses on four specific, measurable, cost-effective activities:

- **G**rowth monitoring which can detect malnutrition before its effects become extreme,
- **O**ral rehydration therapy through a simple solution of salt and sugar as a way to fight diarrheal disease,
- **B**reastfeeding as the most cost-effective way to get nutrition to infants and increase their immune function, and
- **I**mmunizations, which protects children from infectious diseases which might otherwise prove fatal.[40]

Like his colleague Bill Foege, Jim Grant focused UNICEF's efforts on cost-effective, measurable, scalable health interventions—interventions that prevented illnesses and saved lives.[41] And like Bill Foege, Grant was also awarded the Presidential Medal of Freedom—this time by President Bill Clinton in 1994. Influenced by an in-depth Christianization grounded in the medical missions movement of late nineteenth- and early twentieth-century Protestantism, both Foege and Grant represent the response to the secularization of the Social Gospel described by William King as social engineers.

Reconstructionist: the polemics—and faith—of Ivan Illich

Ivan Illich does not strictly fit the mold of King's reconstructionist for the simple fact that he was not a product of Social Gospel Protestantism. I include him here, nonetheless, because his life and work and practice reflect an in-depth Christianization in the reconstructionist mold. Born in Vienna to a Catholic father and a Jewish mother, Illich fled Austria for Italy in 1941 because of his mother's Jewish heritage; most of her family who stayed behind were murdered under Nazi rule.[42] Illich possessed a tremendous intellect—he spoke French, Italian, English, German, Spanish, Croatian, Ancient Greek, Latin, Hindi, and Portuguese—and studied in health sciences (histology), natural sciences (crystallography), philosophy, medieval history, and theology.[43] He was ordained into the Roman Catholic priesthood and served a parish in Washington Heights on Manhattan's far Upper West Side. First as a local parish priest in an immigrant neighborhood and later as a professor in Puerto Rico, he was outspoken in his criticisms of politics—including the ecclesial politics of Catholicism. Further, Illich developed trenchant critiques of modern culture not by diagnosing the common ills we all understand as part and parcel of modern life but by demonstrating the problems with the elements of our societies he called "modern certainties"—education, technology, and health care, to name a few. In *Medical Nemesis*, Illich argued that modern medicine contributed more to illness than to health by reaching past the limits of its capacity to heal; once it reached such a point, the ongoing development and practice of medicine actually exacerbated illness rather than health.

He developed this argument by describing three iatrogenic effects of medicine—clinical, social, and cultural. Iatrogenesis refers to the harm inflicted by medical treatment, a harm that is usually unintended or unforeseen. In contrast to this idea of unintended harm, Illich argued that such harm was entirely predictable in the practice of modern medicine. Clinical iatrogenesis was the direct bodily and material harm caused by medical practice that had reached past the limits of its knowledge. Examples would include the use of a medication to alleviate a symptom but would incur harmful side effects. For Illich, medical experts had the power to carry out clinically iatrogenic medicine only because they had garnered sufficient social authority so that the general public trusted their medical judgments and practices, even when presented with the possibility of ill effects.

Such authority was the result of social iatrogenesis, which Illich described as the medicalization of the ways that modern human beings conceptualize health. In short, we cannot "think" health in our society outside of medicine. The definitions of health, the metrics for measuring it, and the practices for ensuring it are all carried out in the framework of the medical. Medical models were not always the conceptual models we employed to understand health. Prior to the hegemony of medicine, a variety of forms of knowledge contributed to human beings' perceptions of health. These other forms of knowledge were created, sustained, and developed through cultural systems of knowledge (including religion) over and above the medical systems of knowledge that exemplify our modern context. This loss of other ways of knowing about health is the cultural iatrogenesis of medicine.[44]

In 2002, Richard Smith, the editor of the *British Medical Journal*, wrote, "the closest I ever came to a religious experience was listening to Ivan Illich." In a review of the 2002 edition of the text, Smith claimed that

> the power of the book is undiminished [25 years after its initial publication], and its prescience seems remarkable. What was radical in 1974 is in some sense mainstream in 2002. Medicine does seem to have over-reached itself and some reining in will benefit not only patients but also doctors.[45]

Illich did not limit his criticism to medical practice alone. He also argues that public health practice is implicated in the same overreach:

> The level of public health corresponds to the degree to which the means and responsibility for coping with illness are distributed among the total population. This ability to cope can be enhanced but never replaced by medical intervention or by the hygienic characteristics of the environment. That society which can reduce professional intervention to the minimum will provide the best conditions for health . . . A world of optimal and widespread health is obviously a world of minimal and only occasional medical intervention. Healthy people are those who live in healthy homes on a healthy diet in an environment equally fit for birth, growth, work, healing, and dying; they are sustained by a culture that enhances the conscious acceptance of limits to population, of aging, of incomplete recovery and ever-imminent death. Healthy people need minimal bureaucratic interference to mate, give birth, share the human condition, and die . . . The true miracle of modern medicine is diabolical. It consists in making not only individuals but whole populations survive on inhumanly low levels of personal health.[46]

Illich was also deeply critical of development practice outside of global health frameworks, whether sponsored by religious or secular organizations. Illich scolded a 1968 gathering of American students involved in short-term development projects in Mexico, saying:

> In the conversations which I had with you today, I was impressed by two things . . . I was impressed by your insight that the motivation of U.S. volunteers overseas springs mostly from very alienated feelings and concepts. I was equally impressed, by what I interpret as a step forward among would-be volunteers like you: openness to the idea that the only thing you can legitimately volunteer for in Latin America might be voluntary powerlessness, voluntary presence as receivers, as such, as hopefully beloved or adopted ones without any way of returning the gift.
>
> I was equally impressed by the hypocrisy of most of you: by the hypocrisy of the atmosphere prevailing here. I say this as a brother speaking to brothers and sisters . . . Your very insight, your very openness to evaluations of past programs make you hypocrites because you—or at least most of you—have decided to spend this next summer in Mexico, and therefore, you are unwilling to go far enough in your reappraisal of your program. You close your eyes because you want to go ahead and could not do so if you looked at some facts. . . .
>
> Today, the existence of organizations like yours is offensive to Mexico. I wanted to make this statement in order to explain why I feel sick about it all

> and in order to make you aware that good intentions have not much to do with what we are discussing here. To hell with good intentions. This is a theological statement. You will not help anybody by your good intentions.[47]

Illich's iconoclasm led many to assume that he had been de-frocked by the Roman Catholic church. In fact, this is not true. He remained a priest in good-standing throughout his life.[48] And throughout his life, Illich kept articulating his social reconstructionist perspectives, most definitely rejecting any role as a social engineer. In a 1967 speech in Puerto Rico at a conference on Christian Social Relations, Illich was clear in distinguishing between effective and innovative responses to social problems and the particular function of religious faith. He did not denigrate the former but neither did he collapse the latter merely into an instrument to support such responses: "We will need ideological rationalizations for a long time to achieve purposefully planned inventive solutions to social problems. Let consciously secular ideology assume this task. I want to celebrate my faith for no purpose at all."[49]

Through the work of the evangelists, engineers, and reconstructionists, an internationalization of Social Gospel ideals took place through the activities of global health and development. This in-depth Christianization reflected efforts to transfer the empire of the world into global bodies and global initiatives made possible through social critiques and social commitments to a better world for all. The challenges to achieving that vision led to more programs and more critiques as the evangelists, engineers, and reconstructionists began to work more intentionally to build hybrid models that blended the best of each approach. The next chapter explores these blended models.

Notes

1 Robert T. Handy, "The American Religious Depression, 1925–1935." in *Church History* 29, no. 1 (1960): 3. The quote is from the 1939 Presidential Address of the American Society of Church History, given by William Kelley Wright.
2 Ibid., pp. 4–5.
3 William Hocking, *Re-Thinking Missions: A Laymen's Inquiry After One Hundred Years* (New York: Harper & Brothers, 1932), ix.
4 Ibid., p. 19.
5 Ibid., p. 71.
6 Ibid., pp. 199–201.
7 Quoted in Handy, p. 6.
8 Charles Fiske, *The Confessions of a Puzzled Parson* (New York: Charles Scribner, 1928), 14.
9 John Coleman Bennett, "After Liberalism – What?," in *Christian Century* 50 (8 November 1933): 1403.
10 Robert Moats Miller, "The Church Must Go Beyond Modernism: A Faith That Could Not Be Shaken," in *Harry Emerson Fosdick: Preacher, Pastor, Prophet* (New York: Oxford, 1985), 391.
11 Bradley W. Bateman, "Clearing the Ground: The Decline of the Social Gospel and the Rise of Neoclassicism in American Economics," in *History of Political Economy* 30, supplemental volume (1998): 29–52.

12 Thierry Voeltzel, "On religion," in *Religion and Culture: Michel Foucault*, ed. Jeremy Carette (New York: Routledge, 1999), 106–109. Originally published as "La religion," a section from Thierry Voetzel's Ving ans et aprés (Paris: Grasset, 1978).
13 Peter Berger, *The Sacred Canopy: Elements of a Sociological Theory of Religion* (Garden City, NY: Doubleday, 1967), 127.
14 Michel Foucault, "Lecture of 19 February 1975," in *Abnormal: Lectures at the College de France 1974–1975* (New York: Picador, 1999), 177.
15 William McGuire King, "The Emergence of Social Gospel Radicalism: The Methodist Case," in *Church History* 50, No. 4 (1981), 438. King is quoting from the "Statement of Principles and Objectives" of the Fellowship of Socialist Christians.
16 Herbert Welch, "The Church and Social Service," in *Methodist Review* 24, no. 5 (1908): 710–711.
17 King, p. 441.
18 Edwin Earp, *The Social Engineer* (New York: Eaton and Mains, 1911), xiv, 140.
19 King, pp. 442–443. King is quoting George Albert Coe, *The Psychology of Religion* (Chicago: University of Chicago Press, 1916).
20 Ibid., p. 444.
21 The Rockefellers, their relationship to the Social Gospel, and their influence on international secular health and development initiatives were described in some detail in Chapter 3.
22 King, p. 447. The Social Service Bulletin was the monthly journal of the Methodist Federation for Social Service.
23 Ernest Fremont Tittle, *What Must the Church Do to be Saved? And Other Discussions* (New York: Abingdon, 1921), 108.
24 Halford Luccock, "The Resurrection of Jesus Taking Place Today," in *Through the ofYouth*, ed. Halford Luccock and William Reid (New York: Abingdon, 1924), 175.
25 Charles Brent, "The Situation at Home," in *The Foreign Missions Convention at Washington 1925* (New York: Foreign Missions Conference of North America, 1925), 32–33.
26 Robert, p. 53.
27 Harry Emerson Fosdick, *A Christian Conscience About War* (sermon, Geneva Switzerland, September 13, 1925), Online: https://archive.org/details/christianconscie00fosd, accessed February 18, 2018.
28 Walter A. McDougall, *Promised Land, Crusader State: The American Encounter with the World Since 1776* (New York: Houghton Mifflin, 1997), 125.
29 McDougall, p. 125.
30 Unless otherwise cited, the events related to the role of these Protestant leaders on the formation of the United Nations are found in John Nurser, "The 'Ecumenical Movement' Churches, 'Global Order,' and Human Rights: 1938–1948," in *Human Rights Quarterly* 25, no. 4 (2003): 841–881.
31 Nurser, p. 842. The Bretton Woods agreements were established in 1944 in San Francisco and led to the creation of the International Monetary Fund and the World Bank. The citation for the quote by Dulles comes from the meeting minutes of a 1946 meeting in Cambridge, England, on the Conference of the Churches Commission on International Affairs. Those meetings minutes are housed at the World Council of Churches archive and are not searchable online; however, the WCC archive does provide photographic evidence that Dulles was at this meeting.
32 Ibid., p. 845.
33 U.S. Centers for Disease Control and Prevention, *CDC Global Health Strategy, 2012–2105* (Atlanta: U.S. Centers for Disease Control and Prevention, 2012), 11.
34 President Obama made reference to Foege's stint as a medical missionary in his introductory remarks at the ceremony where Foege was awarded the Presidential Medal of Freedom. Foege himself tells the story of his childhood. See William H. Foege, *House on Fire: The Fight to Eradicate Smallpox* (Berkeley, CA: University of California, 2011). The reference to Foege's uncle can be found at Jim Yong Kim, "William H. Foege, Physician: A Lifelong Battle Against Disease," in *U.S. News & World Report* 143, no. 17 (2007), www.usnews.com/news/best-leaders/articles/2007/11/12/william-h-foege, accessed March 11, 2018.
35 Foege, pp. 28–29.

36 In the interest of full disclosure, I want to state as the author of this text that I am also the Acting Director of the Interfaith Health Program that Foege helped found.

37 Kim. Online: www.usnews.com/news/best-leaders/articles/2007/11/12/william-h-foege, accessed March 11, 2018.

38 Mark L. Rosenberg, Elisabeth S. Hayes, Margaret H. McIntyre, and Nancy Neill, *Real Collaboration:What It Takes for Global Health to Succeed* (Berkeley, CA: University of California Press, 2010), 1–2.

39 Kim. Online: www.usnews.com/news/best-leaders/articles/2007/11/12/william-h-foege, accessed March 11, 2018.

40 For further information on UNICEF's GOBI approach, see online: http://rehydrate.org/facts/gobi-fff.htm

41 *New York Times* columnist Nicholas Kristof wrote of Grant that he "launched the child survival revolution with vaccinations and diarrhea treatments that probably saved more lives than were destroyed by Hitler, Mao and Stalin combined."

42 Lee Hoinacki, "The Trajectory of Ivan Illich," in *Bulletin of Science, Technology, and Society* 23, no. 5 (2003): 382.

43 Thierry Pasquot, *Ivan Illich: A Tribute – The Nonconformist* Le Monde Diplomatique, January 2003, 15–19.

44 Ivan Illich, *Medical Nemesis: The Expropriation of Health* (New York: Marion Boyers, 2002 edition).

45 Richard Smith, "Review: 'Limits to Medicine. Medical Nemesis: The Expropriation of Health," in *British Medical Journal* 234 (2002): 923.

46 Illich (2002), Chapter 8, "The Recovery of Health."

47 Ivan Illich, "Yankee, Go Home: The American Do-Gooder in Latin America," in *The Church, Change, and Development* (Chicago: Urban Training Center Press, 1975), 45–46.

48 Lee Hoinacki discusses this misperception among Illich's secular admirers. See pp. 383–384.

49 Ivan Illich, "The Church, Change, and Development," in *The Church, Change, and Development* (Chicago: Urban Training Center Press, 1975), 22.

References

Bateman, Bradley W. "Clearing the Ground: The Decline of the Social Gospel and the Rise of Neoclassicism in American Economics." *History of Political Economy* 30, supplemental volume (1998): 29–52.

Bennett, John Coleman. "After Liberalism—What?" *Christian Century* 50 (8 November 1933): 1403–1406.

Berger, Peter. *The Sacred Canopy: Elements of a Sociological Theory of Religion*. Garden City, NY: Doubleday, 1967.

Brent, Charles. "The Situation at Home." In *The Foreign Missions Convention at Washington 1925*, 27–36. New York: Foreign Missions Conference of North America, 1925.

Fiske, Charles. *The Confessions of a Puzzled Parson*. New York: Charles Scribner, 1928.

Foege, William H. *House on Fire: The Fight to Eradicate Smallpox*. Berkeley, CA: University of California, 2011.

Fosdick, Harry Emerson. "A Christian Conscience About War." Sermon, Geneva, Switzerland, September 13, 1925. https://archive.org/details/christianconscie00fosd. Accessed February 18, 2018.

Foucault, Michel. "Lecture of 19 February 1975," In *Abnormal: Lectures at the College de France 1974–1975*. New York: Picador, 1999.

Handy, Robert T. "The American Religious Depression, 1925–1935." *Church History* 29, no. 1 (1960): 3–16.

Hocking, William. *Re-Thinking Missions: A Laymen's Inquiry After One Hundred Years*. New York: Harper & Brothers, 1932.

Hoinacki, Lee. "The Trajectory of Ivan Illich." *Bulletin of Science, Technology, and Society* 23, no. 5 (2003): 382–389.

Illich, Ivan. *Medical Nemesis: The Expropriation of Health*. New York: Marion Boyers, 2002 edition.

Illich, Ivan. *The Church, Change, and Development*. Chicago: Urban Training Center Press, 1975.

Kim, Jim Yong. "William H. Foege, Physician: A Lifelong Battle Against Disease." *U.S. News & World Report* 143, no. 17 (2007). www.usnews.com/news/best-leaders/articles/2007/11/12/william-h-foege. Accessed March 11, 2018.

King, William McGuire. "The Emergence of Social Gospel Radicalism: The Methodist Case." *Church History* 50, no. 4 (Dec., 1981): 436–449.

Luccock, Halford. "The Resurrection of Jesus Taking Place Today." *Through the of Youth*, ed. Halford Luccock and William Reid, 165–176. New York: Abingdon, 1924.

McDougall, Walter A. *Promised Land, Crusader State: The American Encounter with the World Since 1776*. New York: Houghton Mifflin, 1997.

Miller, Robert Moats. "The Church Must Go Beyond Modernism: A Faith That Could Not Be Shaken." In *Harry Emerson Fosdick: Preacher, Pastor, Prophet*, 389–417. New York: Oxford, 1985.

Nurser, John. "The 'Ecumenical Movement' Churches, 'Global Order,' and Human Rights: 1938–1948." *Human Rights Quarterly* 25, no. 4 (2003): 841–881.

Pasquot, Thierry. "Ivan Illich: A Tribute—The Nonconformist." In *Le Monde Diplomatique*, 15–19, January 2003.

Rosenberg, Mark L., Elisabeth S. Hayes, Margaret H. McIntyre, and Nancy Neill. *Real Collaboration: What It Takes for Global Health to Succeed*. Berkeley, CA: University of California Press, 2010.

Smith, Richard. "Review: 'Limits to Medicine. Medical Nemesis: The Expropriation of Health." *British Medical Journal* 234 (2002): 923.

Tittle, Ernest Fremont. *What Must the Church Do to be Saved? And Other Discussions*. New York: Abingdon, 1921.

U.S. Centers for Disease Control and Prevention. *CDC Global Health Strategy, 2012- 2105*. Atlanta: U.S. Centers for Disease Control and Prevention, 2012.

Voeltzel, Thierry. "On religion." In *Religion and Culture: Michel Foucault*, ed. Jeremy, Carette. New York: Routledge, 1999.

Welch, Herbert. "The Church and Social Service." *Methodist Review* 24, no 5 (1908): 707–715.

5 Blurring the lines between evangelists, engineers, and reconstructionists

The last chapter developed an argument first articulated by William Mcguire King regarding the ways in which the Social Gospel movement of American Protestantism dissolved by the end of the Second World War. However, rather than a dissolution into nothing, the chapter argued that this dissolution had the characterization of an in-depth Christianization in which the principles of the Social Gospel informed a variety of institutions responsible for today's global health and development initiatives. King described the work of the Social Gospel being carried forth by three actors after its dissolution: social evangelists, social engineers, and social reconstructionists.[1] This chapter examines the ways in which these three movements have combined to influence global health and development practice for the last 50 years.

Evangelist/engineer

In the 1960s and 1970s, Protestant Christians in Europe and North America were struggling to articulate a new model of health ministries. A number of changes had upended the way in which medical missions had been carried out: many of the faith-based health facilities founded by American and European missionaries over the past 60 years had been transferred to in-country organizations and were no longer managed by those missionary bodies; other mission health facilities had been nationalized by the governments of newly independent nations as they threw off the colonial rule under the nations from which those same missionaries had come; falling membership among liberal Protestants in both North America and Europe left those denominations with fewer resources to devote to medical missions even as mission models among more conservative Christian traditions that focused on converting populations to the Christian faith began gaining ground, and the development of governmental health systems had created a crisis among the leadership of those faith-based facilities who faced challenges in funding and care to the poor. The idea of medical care as an indispensable element of foreign missions—an idea which had been so central to Protestant understandings of the missionary endeavor for the first half of the century—could no longer be carried out in the same way.

In 1964, Protestants gathered in Tübingen, Germany under the leadership of the Deutsches Institut für Ärztliche Mission (DIFAEM)—or the German Institute for Medical Mission to look at these challenges. Participants at the Tübingen consultation struggled to articulate a new understanding of the church's mission in relation to health. The statement that was fashioned as one output of the meeting reflected a number of changes to such an understanding. First, the focus shifted from medical care for those who were sick to broader programs in support of health for all. The consultation certainly reflected on medical missions and the role of faith-based facilities in providing medical care in most parts of the world but participants also articulated a broader concept of health and described health initiatives outside of medical facilities that contributed to health. Second, this shift in the conceptualization in health required a shift in understanding how health ministries were carried out that highlighted the roles, responsibilities, and contributions not only of stand-alone health facilities but of every local congregation. Third, it noted that the bulk of medical care provided by faith-based facilities in low- and middle-income countries was provided not by facilities owned or managed by European and North American missionary organizations but by in-country denominational bodies, many of which struggled to keep facilities operating in light of the various demands they faced as their nations emerged from colonial rule.[2]

The Tübingen consultation was one of the catalysts for the formation of the Christian Medical Commission (CMC) of the World Council of Churches (WCC) in 1968,[3] although the CMC was initially more narrowly focused on medical care than on broader health ministries. The reasons for this are twofold. First, the WCC was committed to supporting denominational partners representing the new nations that had thrown off colonial rule in the 1950s and 1960s and these denominations were already taxed with a number of pressing needs. As a result, the administration of health facilities was not a high priority in the countries and the WCC allocated resources for providing administrative, fiscal, and technical support to fill the gap; these support efforts were an early focus of the CMC, despite the broader conceptualization of health that had come out of Tübingen. Second, there were concerns that a general focus on health would provide too large of a voice to denominational partners within the WCC who were critical of clinical medicine and championed faith healing. In fact, the WCC intentionally chose the name Christian Medical Commission over the phrase Christian Health Commission:

> when the original proposal to create a Christian Health Commission was announced it attracted an immediate response from various spiritual and divine healing groups which felt that, at last, they were being provided a forum within a worldwide ecumenical body. Since the Commission was intended to

> assist the churches which were engaged in medical services around the world it was decided that it would be more appropriate to designate it as such.[4]

Socrates Litsios served as a senior scientist at the WHO for over 20 years. He described the formative role of the CMC played in establishing primary health care as a priority within the WHO. For Litsios, the impact of the 1964 Tübingen consultation went beyond the key findings named above. Quoting from the Tübingen I report, Litsios argued that:

> The medicalization of the healing art had led to a rift between the work of "those with specialized medical training and the life of the congregation." The entire congregation had a part to play in healing.
>
> "The consultation made a strong case that modern medical care was at odds with the quest for health and wholeness. The hospital had become a "factory for repair," in which the patient had been broken down into "pathological parts." The "results of a battery of tests" were more important "than the relationship of persons in a therapeutic encounter.
>
> [This] concept of wholeness and health had strong implications for the congregation, a position that had emerged from Tübingen I. It is only "when the Christian community serves the sick person in its midst [that] it becomes itself healed and whole." Going further, [the report] argued that the healing congregation accepts the fact "that any one individual group or nation may not be entitled to an unlimited use of the resources of healing when such unlimited use will mean less available resources of healing for others."[23] Thus, [the report's] argument suggested a moral basis for individuals and communities to be involved in any consideration of how resources are to be used to promote their health.[5]

In short, Tübingen was critical in helping the commission make the case to the WCC to broaden its focus to include not only medical facilities but also to support the development of curative and preventive services to the larger community through local congregations.

Over the next few years, the WCC launched or helped replicate a number of holistic health initiatives. When Halfdan Mahler became Director General of the WHO in 1973, he sought to tear down the siloed approach to health initiatives that had characterized the organization in its prior years. The emerging model of primary health care consisted of multi-sectoral approaches to health that sought input from local communities regarding their needs, priorities, and own resources in relation to health and illness. The concept revolutionized the technocratic model that had come before and the local congregation initiatives identified by the CMC represented some of the most promising and effective examples of this model. In 1974, the WHO and the WCC through the CMC entered into a memorandum of understanding characterized by "joint involvement in common endeavors on a very practical level." Through this memorandum, the WCC had a voice on health policies and priorities at the annual WHO Assembly and on the Executive Board, the first non-governmental actor from the faith-based sector to wield such influence just as the CCIA had done in contributing to the UN Charter almost thirty years before.[6]

The Tübingen Consultation and the Christian Medical Commission are examples of the social evangelists and social engineers working together to articulate a new model of health ministry informed by theological commitments and made possible by understanding feasible, cost-effective models that could be implemented and replicated as part of a broader approach to global health and development.

Evangelist/reconstructionist

The partnerships built between American Protestants and Protestants in Europe in the middle decades of the twentieth century through the channels of the United Nations and the World Council of Churches led not only to internationalization of medical missions' initiatives; there were other effects as well. Over time, America's Protestant leaders—often because of the influence of foreign missions programs—recognized the insights that religious leaders from other parts of the world offered based on their own experiences and contexts. These leaders contributed to new theological perspectives that offered trenchant and often radical critiques during the independence movements of various nations to emerge from European colonial rule. In South Africa, for example, theologies and programs of resistance toward the Apartheid system of racial segregation and government helped provide a moral grounding for social mobilization to resist and eventually overthrow and dismantle the government.[7] Similar critiques of colonialism and post-colonial articulations of alternatives occurred across other African nations.[8]

Critiques from these movements were not limited to European powers. America's manipulations of poorer societies in its seemingly endless chess game with Soviet Russia were also a target of strong theological critiques[9] and of organized movements within civil societies.[10] These theologies criticized America's military and defense policies, but they also called health and development implementers to task for enabling foreign assistance to become a strategic instrument in America's own self interests. Secular movements informed by critiques from thinkers such as Paolo Freire influenced religious initiatives and theological perspectives—most notably from liberation theologies first voiced by Roman Catholic communities and then by Protestant communities in Central and South America, sub-Saharan Africa, and southern and eastern Asia.[11] Globally, Protestant Christians organized and agitated for nuclear disarmament, an end to the Cold War, peace movements, feminist movements, the American civil rights movements for Black Americans, and economic justice movements. These movements contributed to Han theologies from south Asia, mujerista theologies from Central and South America,[12] and African theologies from groups such as the Circle of Concerned African Women Theologians.[13]

In the United States, there were theological movements that echoed these global contexts. First- and second-wave feminist theologians articulated strong critiques of the patriarchal structures and practices of Christian communities and institutions.[14] African American Christians articulated Black theologies,[15] and when African American women decided that such theologies failed to address the sexism of Black men, they developed womanist theologies that offered critiques of aspects of Black theologies and feminist theologies even as they expressed solidarity with core elements in each of those genres.[16] Lesbian and gay people—often writing as laypeople because Christian communities refused to ordain them—developed gay theologies and later queer theologies.[17] These movements were not just incubators of theological texts; they influenced practices of faith so that marching in an anti-war rally or participating in a consciousness raising group on sexism and racism was part of community ministry or Christian education in some churches.

Liberal Protestants were active in the civil rights movement of the 1960s and Riverside Church in the City of New York—that bastion of liberal Protestantism described by the *New York Times* as "the Vatican of America's mainstream Protestants"—invited Martin Luther King, Jr. and other civil rights leaders to preach. Reverend King wrote a long note to Riverside's pastor Harry Emerson Fosdick on the flyleaf of his book *Stride Toward Freedom*, a book which detailed the Montgomery bus boycotts. The note read:

> If l were called upon to select the greatest preacher of this century, I would choose your name. If I were called upon to select the foremost prophets of our generation, I would choose you to head this list. If I were called upon to select the Christian saints of our day, again I would have to place you on the list. Because of all these things and the inspiration you've been to me, I present you this book.

And yet, there were also significant tensions at Riverside, emblematic of tensions between predominantly white, mainline Protestant leaders and congregations and black civil rights leaders. In 1969, James Foreman, a leader in the Student Non-Violent Coordinating Committee and in the Black Panther political party, interrupted Sunday worship at Riverside by marching into the pulpit with six colleagues to demand $500 million from America's white churches as reparation payment for the legacy of slavery and racism in America. Riverside did not pay—Rockefeller's endowment was not that large—but it did agree to donate a portion of the earnings from that endowment to civil rights and anti-poverty movements.

Public health and race in 1960s America

In 1965, the U.S. Department of Labor issued a report entitled *The Negro Family: The Case for National Action* which detailed the social and economic disparities facing African American families. Daniel Moynihan, the Assistant Secretary of the Department of Labor, authored the piece, which came to be known as the Moynihan Report. Moynihan, who would later serve four terms as U.S. Senator representing New York, had drafted the commencement address that President Lyndon Johnson had given at Howard University, a historically black university in Washington, DC. Johnson's speech was warmly received by black leaders. Martin Luther King told Johnson that "never before has a president articulated the depths and dimensions of the problem of racial injustice more eloquently and profoundly."[18] The themes outlined in Johnson's speech—social and economic disparities between black and white Americans, generational cycles of poverty, urban decay, and family breakdown—were in many ways the same issues explored in the Moynihan report.

Despite the generally positive reception of Johnson's commencement address and the fact that the report that followed only a few months later echoed the same themes as those in that speech, the Moynihan report generated controversy from the moment it was published. The report focused on the social costs of single-family systems in African American communities:

> In essence, the Negro community has been forced into a matriarchal structure which, because it is so out of line with the rest of the American society, seriously retards the progress of the group as a whole, and imposes a crushing burden on the Negro male and, in consequence, on a great many Negro women as well.[19]

Religious leaders with the National Council of Churches offered some of the most strident critiques, taking the report to task for its pathological portrayal of too many Black families led by single mothers with no active involvement by fathers. Benjamin Payton, director of the Office of Church and Race of the Protestant Council of New York City, penned an article in the Christian magazine *Christianity and Crisis*, arguing that Moynihan mischaracterized Black communities by focusing on limited and misinterpreted data to paint a pathological picture when, in fact, those communities displayed tremendous resiliency:

> the student movement, the continued power of the Negro church and the tremendous "coping skills" generated by the Negro family itself are but a few of the factors that demonstrate the community's great reserves of untapped power and health. If these were harnessed under Negro leadership but with larger and more relevant national resources and co-operation, the remaining

> gap between Negroes and whites—a gap caused by continuing forms of discrimination—can be rapidly closed.[20]

Payton went on the lead the Commission on Religion and Race in the National Council of Churches. In 1966, as Director of the Commission, he authored an essay entitled "Black Power." To get the document published and in front of the widest possible audience the NCC paid for a full-page ad in *The New York Times* on July 31 that was, in fact, the content of Payton's essay.[21] Over 150 Protestant leaders were signatories to the document. "Black Power" became a touchpoint in the Black theology movement that has played such a central role in liberal Christian theological writing for the past 50 years. Gayraud Wilmore, a leading voice in the Black theology tradition, said that the July 1966 article was "the beginning of Black reflection on the racial situation in America independent of the White theologians and ethicists. Thus it was one starting point for a separate Black theology."[22]

In his social history of the Moynihan Report. Daniel Geary describes Payton's role in this way:

> Payton challenged the technocratic nature of Moynihan's liberalism by advocating the democratic participation of ordinary individuals. To Payton, the Moynihan Report embodied how out of touch policy-makers were. "The important moral issue at stake," Payton asserted, "is whether social experts can relate to private citizens as persons or merely as objects." Payton voiced a growing discontent with how white liberals had dominated racial discourse . . . and claimed that white liberals were "unable to appreciate the need for local community action on the part of Negroes themselves." They saw African Americans not as agents in their own right but as objects to "be acted upon, by the social experts, the federal government, and patron benefactors."

Benjamin Payton was a theologian, activist, foundation administrator, and university president. His focus was not public health. Nonetheless, his criticisms of the Moynihan Report highlighted aspects of public health practice in the United States that others critiqued: an uncritical use of data; failure to account for one's own social location and influences even while analyzing the social forces at work in other communities; and a reliance on technical knowledge over the insights, wisdom, and capacities of local communities that are the subject of the public health practitioner's concern. Over 30 years after his leadership with the NCC, Payton served as President of Tuskegee University. In that capacity on May 16, 1997, Payton was at the White House as an official guest to hear President Clinton offer a formal apology on behalf of the United States for the syphilis study conducted by the United States Public Health Service in and around Tuskegee, Alabama.

The study, which lasted for over 40 years from the 1932–1972, enrolled 600 black men in a longitudinal trial to understand the long-term effects of untreated syphilis. Three hundred and ninety-nine of the study subjects were men infected with syphilis; they were never offered any treatment, even after effective treatment with penicillin became available in 1947.

At the White House event, President Clinton offered these words to the surviving men enrolled in the study, the family members of study participants, and members of the Tuskegee community, including Benjamin Payton:

> The people who ran the study at Tuskegee diminished the stature of man by abandoning the most basic ethical precepts. They forgot their pledge to heal and repair. They had the power to heal the survivors and all the others and they did not. Today, all we can do is apologize. But you have the power, for only you—Mr. Shaw, the others who are here, the family members who are with us in Tuskegee—only you have the power to forgive. Your presence here shows us that you have chosen a better path than your government did so long ago. You have not withheld the power to forgive. I hope today and tomorrow every American will remember your lesson and live by it.[23]

The syphilis study in Macon County, Alabama mirrored in many ways another research initiative carried out by the USPHS. This work occurred in Guatemala. From 1946–1948, the USPHS worked in collaboration with the Pan American Health Sanitary Bureau (now the Pan American Health Organization, a regional body of the World Health Organization) and the Government of Guatemala to study whether penicillin could be used as a prophylaxis against syphilis infection and not only as a treatment once infected. In order to ascertain the prophylactic effects of penicillin, the study required exposing participants to syphilis. U.S. Public Health Service staff developed a design that enrolled prisoners as study participants: 696 men who were serving sentences in Guatemalan prisons. Prisons gave their permission for the study but neither the men involved nor their families were informed. To expose the men to syphilis, the study recruited sex workers who had tested positive for the infection and offered the men in the study the chance to have sex with the sex workers as a means of infecting them.

Dr. John Cutler, the Public Health Service officer who coordinated the study in Guatemala and also worked in Tuskegee for two different periods of time, was aware that the study failed to meet basic ethics standards. In 1947, a short article in the *New York Times* noted that syphilis transmission had been prevented in animal studies involving rabbits but noted that the results may not hold in humans and that "it would be necessary to shoot living syphilis germs into human bodies . . . Since this is ethically impossible, it may take years to gather the information needed." Cutler saw the article in the *Times* and wrote to Dr. John Mahoney, director of the USPHS' Venereal Disease Research Lab (VDRL) in New York to remind him that a VDRL study was doing precisely what the *Times* article had deemed impossible—infecting humans with living syphilis germs. In ongoing correspondence, Mahoney and Cutler decided that keeping the study secret was essential, as noted in Cutler's communication:

> It is becoming just as clear to us as it appears to be to you that it would not be advisable to have too many people concerned with this work in order to keep down talk and premature writing. I hope that it would be possible to keep the work strictly in your hands without necessity for outside advisors or workers other than those who fit into your program and who can be trusted not to talk. We are just a little bit concerned about the possibility of having anything said about our program that would adversely affect its continuation.[24]

In 2010, Cornell West, one of the leading Christian thinkers in America on race, culture, and politics, spoke to the national meeting of the American Public Health Association. West spoke in a plenary session that specifically addressed the effects of racism on public health and examined the legacy costs of the Tuskegee study. The connection to the violence carried out in Guatemala was not yet public. West's words represent an evangelist/reconstructionist bridging as a way of providing a theological message in the context of racism, politics, and power. This is a portion of West's speech:

> Being willing to tell the truth is to allow suffering to speak . . . So the fundamental question in talking about justice is what kind of human being will you choose to be? What kind of virtues, what kind of character, what kind of values do you want to exemplify in your life? . . .
>
> 40% of black and brown children living in poverty, 20% of all of America's precious children living in poverty in the richest nation in the history of the world. That's a moral disgrace. That's an ethical abomination . . . 4/5 of all the income between 1980 and 2005 went to the top 1%. And then when it comes to working on poor people's education our leaders tell us that we don't have the money. What about poor people who need quality health, quality education? . . .
>
> Some of us come out of the legacy of Martin Luther King, Jr. and we are unapologetic about it. Which means that we know that there's a connection between questioning and deep giving and loving. I use the word love explicitly because love is a steadfast commitment to the wellbeing of others. I also speak as a Christian . . . I learn from my atheist and agnostic and Buddhist and Judaic brothers and sisters. But what I bring to the table has to do with this legacy of love. . . .
>
> We don't accept that the whole terrain has to be shaped in such a way that poor people and working people generation after generation after generation experience social neglect rather than social justice, social abandonment rather than social justice . . . When I run into people who are optimistic in America,

> I know that individually they're doing well but they have forgotten their fellow citizens who are catching hell. We're in this together. We hang together. We're going to be prisoners of hope, we're going to be veterans of hope. We're going to be ambassadors of hope, which means we decide to be human beings in such a way that we think critically against the grain, that prophetically we're going to bear witness to justice motivated by a deep compassion . . . I'm going to allow my light to shine because I'm a member of the American Public Health Association.[25]

Religious responses to HIV

When the first cases of an unknown but deadly illness were reported in the United States in 1981, medical doctors were stymied. They did not know the cause of the odd and rarely-seen infections and they marveled at the inaction of patients' immune systems in fighting it. HIV, the virus that slowly depletes the immune system of those infected to the point that they can no longer fight off pathogens, would not be identified for another four years as the causative organism behind this immune system failure. In the interim, that broad variety of opportunistic infections showing up in the bodies of those with compromised immune systems took on a variety of different names, before AIDS—Acquired Immune Deficiency Syndrome—gained widespread acceptance. One early and informal acronym was WOGS, or Wrath of God Syndrome.[26] HIV and religion have been intertwined because HIV is one of a special subset of diseases which elicit moral judgments. This is not the case with many diseases—diabetes, for example, does not result in strong and sometimes contentious moral pronouncements—but because it is an infectious disease spread through intimate practices such as sex or drug use, HIV carries with it a series of competing moral positions. Though it is not the sole driver of these moral positions, religion is clearly a powerful force.

The World Council of Churches first developed a formal response to the HIV epidemic in 1986. The document *AIDS and the Churches* included medical information; theological perspectives; a call for churches to offer compassionate care, education and prevention programs; and models for compassionate social ministry. The Executive Committee also included the following points in the document:

- to confess that churches as institutions have been slow to speak and to act, that many Christians have been quick to judge and condemn many of the people who have fallen prey to the disease; and that through their silence, many churches share responsibility for the fear that has swept our world more quickly than the virus itself.
- to affirm and support the entire medical and research community in its efforts to combat the disease.
- to affirm that God deals with us in love and mercy and that we are therefore freed from simplistic moralizing about those who are attacked by the virus.[27]

It took 15 more years for the WCC to integrate an ongoing, targeted response to HIV into its programs, launching a funded initiative under the auspices of the WCC in 2001 called the Ecumenical HIV/AIDS Initiatives and Advocacy (EHAIA).[28] EHAIA, which still exists today, works to address HIV-related stigma and equip local churches to respond to the epidemic. To complement EHAIA's efforts, the WCC also supports a number of HIV advocacy efforts through the Ecumenical Advocacy Alliance[29] and publishes resource materials.[30]

Another religious body to respond to the global HIV epidemic is INERELA+, the International Network of Religious Leaders Living with or Affected by HIV/AIDS. In 1992, the Reverend Canon Gideon Byamugisha, an Anglican priest from Uganda publicly disclosed his HIV status. Many of Gideon's supporters and friends gathered at a retreat in 2002 to mark the ten years of ministry made possible by his decision to identify himself as a priest living with HIV. Participants in that retreat decided to start a new religious organization to fight HIV-related stigma. At first, the organization worked only across sub-Saharan Africa but it has since grown to encompass 19 national chapters in Africa, Asia, Latin America, and North America as a global office which individuals can also join. Today, INERELA+ includes over 10,000 members from a variety of faith traditions.

INERELA+ advocates in local, global, and regional contexts to lower stigma and build commitments with religious leaders to address the HIV epidemic. INERELA+ focuses its efforts on fighting stigma, shame, discrimination, denial, inaction, and misaction through four commitments it identifies as its SAVE model: **S**afer practices, **A**ccess to treatment, **V**oluntary counseling and testing, and **E**mpowerment. INERELA+ clearly addresses HIV-related stigma from within religious traditions and offers a platform for those who are often stigmatized and silenced to speak. In this way, it is one of the few religious groups to encourage difficult discussions on sensitive topics such as sex work, drug use, and homosexuality and to ensure that when those discussions take place that the insights and opinions of those directly affected are heard. INERELA+ has programs in the areas of sexual and reproductive health, including adolescent sexual health; gender justice and gender-based violence; sexual diversity that affirms lesbian, gay, bisexual, transgender, intersexed, and queer people; and transformative masculinities to bring men and boys into coordinated, sustained HIV responses in local congregations and communities.[31]

All of these examples reflect a bridging of the social evangelist and the social reconstructionist. Whether we consider Payton's critiques in the 1960s as a staff member of the NCC, Cornell West's words to the American Public Health Association, the myriad theologies that have been developed by women and men from various parts of the world who have articulated critiques of social and political systems from the context of their Christian faith, or programs to address HIV and lower stigma in religious communities, we can see in all of those responses a strong prophetic voice employed by a reconstructionist to articulate a message of good news as an evangelist. Such efforts demonstrate an in-depth Christianization of a Social Gospel that has become secularized.

Engineer/reconstructionist

Perhaps the hardest bridge to build between King's three actors is the one from engineer to reconstructionist. Engineers reflect the value of evidence and technical capacities to solve complex problems. Reconstructionists adopt critical attitudes toward an institution or a practice. Trying to develop evidence-based models and technical capacities while also critically reflecting on the processes by which they were developed is nearly impossible. But there are a few instances.

From 1973 to 1988, Halfdan Mahler served as the third Director General of the World Health Organization. At the time Mahler assumed leadership of the WHO, the organization had for over twenty years been focused on specific infectious diseases such as malaria. This vertical approach in which outsider experts assessed particular aspects of the disease (for example, the vectors of transmission) was the hallmark of the WHO's approach to global health. Mahler, more than any other person within the body, was responsible for a wholesale shift in priorities that focused not on the technical expertise of outsiders coming in to a foreign country and culture to intervene but on the health capacities and resources of local communities to set their own health priorities in partnership with outsiders who could offer assistance and increase capacity when requested. The primary health care model—a model that was, in part, envisioned through the work of the Christian Medical Commission and the Tübingen consultation described above—represented this shift. Speaking to the 30th World Health Assembly in 1977, Mahler made his case for this shift:

> Essential health care requires essential health technology, a technology which people can understand and which the non-expert can apply. The identification or generation of such technology forms part of the revolution in community health and thus presents a tremendous challenge to the World Health Organization. We just cannot afford to continue the indiscriminate use of methods, machines and medicines, so many of which have never undergone the critical evaluation of a controlled trial let alone a proper cost /effectiveness analysis. If this applies to primary health care—in which, let me say, I include such environmental health measures as the provision of drinking—water and waste disposal—it certainly also applies to the other tiers of the health care system.
>
> In an era when such dramatic and productive efforts have been made to rid ourselves of political colonialism, it is unthinkable that we should continue to tolerate technological neo- colonialism in health. We must break the chains of dependence on unproved, over-sophisticated and over-costly health

> technology by developing another kind of technology that is more appropriate because it is technically sound, culturally acceptable and financially feasible. The Organization has launched a programme that will focus first of all on the technology appropriate for primary health care, but which will certainly have to deal in the course of time with all the other aspects of health care.
>
> You will appreciate the enormous professional, commercial and therefore political implications of such a programme of appropriate health technology, for we may often find ourselves in opposition to the medical and allied professions and industries. To succeed, we shall need to work together more than ever before, whatever our professional expertise, not only to generate new technologies, but also to prove their worth as compared with the conventional ones.[32]

As the son of a Danish Baptist preacher, Mahler considered becoming a Protestant pastor during his adolescence. At 15, he began preaching but finally opted for a career in medicine, and from there in global health. If Mahler retained any religious devotion into his adulthood, he expressed rarely in public contexts. While he may not have represented a Social Gospel evangelist, he did nonetheless become a strong advocate for critical reassessments of "business-as-usual" for the WHO's structures and practices. In this way, he bridged an engineer/reconstructionist approach. Further, his decision to establish formal collaboration with the Christian Medical Commission of the World Council of Churches set the ground for a rare instance of shared participation among the evangelists, engineers, and reconstructionists at a macro-level far beyond those found in local communities. This holistic model was reflected in the Alma-Ata Conference on Primary Health Care in 1978.

Evangelist/engineer/reconstructionist

In the fall of 1978, various leaders in global health and development met in Alma-Ata, the capital and largest city in the Kazakh state in the Soviet Union. The meeting, convened by the World Health Organization (WHO) was designed to map the way forward in the full adoption of primary health care as a global health strategy. Primary health care has three focuses: 1) local communities set the priorities for health and development programs based on their own interests, 2) macro-level actors from the government and civil society should support health and development initiatives by strengthening the capacity and resources that already exists in local communities rather than by implementing a stand-alone program administered by outsider experts in the field, and 3) progress in health and development is achieved not only through the formal initiatives of health and development organizations but primarily through community-led activities that work to improve health through prevention and address the social forces that create health and economic disparities in the first place.

Since 1974, the WHO had been working to implement primary health care into all of its programs and had looked to the CMC of the World Council of Churches for examples of successful primary health care programs that already existed. The CMC had a formal memorandum with the WHO to work together on health and development initiatives of common interest—these initiatives focused on primary health care. In many ways, the Alma-Ata conference represented the culmination of these efforts. There were 535 delegates representing 135 countries. Staff from seven UN agencies also participated, along with 62 representatives from civil society. Of the civil society, the largest constituency came from religious bodies, which included the CMC, the International Committee of Catholic Nurses, Baha'i International, the Baptist World Alliance, the Aga Khan Health Boards, Caritas Internationalis, and the Friends World Committee for Consultation.[33] Conference delegates crafted a declaration that was revolutionary in its tone:

> The Conference strongly reaffirms that health . . . is a fundamental human right and that the attainment of the highest possible level of health is a most important world-wide social goal whose realization requires the action of many other social and economic sectors in addition to the health sector.
>
> The existing gross inequality in the health status of the people particularly between developed and developing countries . . . is politically, socially and economically unacceptable and is, therefore, of common concern to all countries. Economic and social development, based on a New International Economic Order, is of basic importance to the fullest attainment of health for all and to the reduction of the gap between the health status of the developing and developed countries. . . .
>
> Governments have a responsibility for the health of their people which can be fulfilled only by the provision of adequate health and social measures. A main social target . . . should be the attainment by all peoples of the world by the year 2000 of a level of health that will permit them to lead a socially and economically productive life. Primary healthcare is the key to attaining this target as part of development in the spirit of social justice.
>
> An acceptable level of health for all the people of the world by the year 2000 can be attained through a fuller and better use of the world's resources, a considerable part of which is now spent on armaments and military conflicts. A genuine policy of independence, peace, détente and disarmament could and should release additional resources that could well be devoted to peaceful aims and in particular to the acceleration of social and economic development of which primary health care, as an essential part, should be allotted its proper share.
>
> The International Conference on Primary Health Care calls for urgent and effective national and international action to develop and implement primary health care throughout the world and particularly in developing countries in a

> spirit of technical cooperation and in keeping with a New International Economic Order.[34]

In the fall of 1978, hundreds of the leading health officials from across the globe committed to a fundamental change in how health and development were understood and services were carried out. Technical interventions carried out by outside experts would take a back seat to community initiatives that challenged the social, economic, political, and cultural forces contributing to and sustaining health and economic disparities. Delegates committed to fundamental structural changes in governmental and economic systems at the highest level, affirming the principles of a New International Economic Order championed by the United Nations that would institute economic programs and policies designed to benefit developing nations even if wealthier nations faced economic headwinds as a result.[35] All of the principles outlined in the Alma-Ata declaration were truly revolutionary and leaders from most of the world's nations—including all of the leading economic and political powers—committed to them in the fall of 1978.

What happened to this revolution? What thwarted it? The answers to such questions require us to look at the broader social-political context in the late 1970s and early 1980s. American and Great Britain elected Ronald Reagan and Margaret Thatcher, both of whom were strong advocates of free market capitalism and had little appetite for New Economic International Orders. In fact, these shifting political-economic priorities led to new global priorities for addressing the debt burden of emerging nations. The Bretton Woods institutions implemented structural adjustment policies that were diametrically opposed to the macro-level economic reforms called for at Alma-Ata. A social reconstructionist vision took a back seat to a much less ambitious approach called selective primary health care that many social engineers would love.

In fact, the global immunization campaign championed by Grant (at UNICEF) and Foege (at the Taskforce for Child Survival) was a cornerstone of the selective primary health care model. This is not to say anything about the respective positions of either Grant or Foege on economic policies such as structural adjustment or on the more revolutionary vision of Alma-Ata. Nonetheless, the limitations of actually implementing the vision of Alma-Ata in practice highlight the challenges of carrying out reconstructionist commitments at a societal level. This doesn't mean we give up trying; rather, it reminds us of the need for clear-eyed analysis of the social and political forces at play.

In an interview with the *Bulletin of the World Health Organization*, Mahler, that son of the strict Baptist preacher, invoked religious and spiritual language as he reflected nostalgically on the primary health care movement to which he had committed himself 30 years earlier:

> The 1970s was a warm decade for social justice. That's why after Alma-Ata in 1978, everything seemed possible. Then came an abrupt reversal, when the

International Monetary Fund (IMF) promoted the Structural Adjustment Program with all kinds of privatization, and that drew skepticism towards the Alma-Ata consensus and weakened commitment to the primary health care strategy. WHO regions kept on fighting in countries, but there was no support from the World Bank and the IMF. And the biggest disappointment was when some United Nations agencies switched to a "selective" approach to primary health care. That brought us right back to square one. We had started with selective health-care programmes, single diseases such as malaria and tuberculosis in the 1950s and 1960s. Then we had this spiritual and intellectual awakening that came out of Alma-Ata, and suddenly some proponents of primary health care went back to the old selective approach again. Perhaps, paradoxically, Alma-Ata had in such instances the opposite effect to the one intended, as it made people think too much about selection, rather than following the Alma-Ata gospel of health for all.[36]

In that interview, Mahler may have sounded like a social evangelist; in his address to the World Health Assembly in 2008, he sounded like a reconstructionist and seemed quite capable of channeling the fiery rhetoric of the preacher:

> Unless we all become partisans in renewed local and global battles for social and economic equity in the spirit of distributive justice, we shall indeed betray the future of our children and grandchildren. My memory tells me that the World Health Assembly had this in mind when, in 1977, it decided that the main social target for governments and WHO in the coming decades should be the attainment of what is known as "Health for All" . . . That is, I believe as it should be. When people are mere pawns in an economic and profit growth game, that game is mostly lost for the underprivileged. . . .
>
> Are you ready to address yourselves seriously to the existing gap between the health "haves" and the health "have-nots" and to adopt concrete measures to reduce it? . . . Are you ready to make preferential allocations of health resources to the social periphery as an absolute priority?
>
> Are you ready to mobilize and enlighten individuals, families and communities in order to ensure their full identification with primary health care, their participation in its planning and management and their contribution to its application? . . . Are you ready to introduce, if necessary, radical changes in the existing health delivery system so that it properly supports primary health care as the overriding health priority?
>
> Are you ready to fight the political and technical battles required to overcome any social and economic obstacles and professional resistance to the universal introduction of primary health care?
>
> Alma-Ata was, in my biased opinion, one of the rare occasions where a sublime consensus between the haves and the have-nots in local and global health emerged . . . In conclusion, my personal view is that the Alma-Ata primary

> health care consensus has had major inspirational and operational impacts in many countries having a critical mass of political and professional leadership combined with adequate human and financial resources to test its adaptability and applicability within the local realities through a heavy dose of systems and operations research.[37]

A budding global health and development framework began to emerge in the middle decades of the twentieth century. While there were undoubtedly various forces that helped fashion this framework, it is nonetheless the case that the evangelistic, engineering, and reconstructionist commitments of those who supported Social Gospel principles in the mission of an in-depth Christianization were significant forces in such efforts. In these ways, they were working to carry out the second phase of the transfer of empire. If American Christians up through the early twentieth century had seen their nation as the culmination of God's intention for the government of the world, there was in these efforts at internationalization and comfort with secularization a vision to see the transfer of the empire of the world disperse from the United States to other nations and other systems. But American Christianity was engaged not only in these types of efforts during these decades. As tensions between America and Russia coalesced into the Cold War, Christianity became a means to articulate a civil religion in America. The complex and uneasy relationship between American Protestantism and Cold War politics is the subject of the next chapter.

Notes

1 William McGuire King, "The Emergence of Social Gospel Radicalism: The Methodist Case," in *Church History* 50, no. 4 (1981): 436–449.

2 "The Beginning – Tübingen I, 1964" in *Contact*, Special Series, no. 2 (1979):1–6. Contact is the magazine of the Christian Medical Commission of the World Council of Churches. This chapter in the special edition of Contact Magazine contains the conclusions of the 1964 in a section entitled "Statement of Tübingen I." See also, Christopher H. Grundmann, "The Legacy of Tübingen I," in *Christian Responses to Health and Development: Symposium at the German Institute for Medical Mission (DIFAEM)*, pp. 12–25 (Tübingen: DIFAEM, 2014), 18–19.

3 Isabel Apawo Phiri, "The Healing Ministry of the Churches Today," in *Christian Responses to Health and Development: Symposium at the German Institute for Medical Mission (DIFAEM)*, pp. 5–11 (Tübingen: DIFAEM, 2014), 5

4 James McGilvray, *The Quest for Health and Wholeness* (Tübingen, The German Institute for Medical Mission, 1981). McGilvray served as the first director of the CMC.

5 Socrates Litsios, "The Christian Medical Commission and the Development of the World Health Organizations Primary Health Care Approach," in *American Journal of Public Health* 94, no. 11 (2004): 1887.

6 Phiri, p. 6.

7 A catalyst in the movement was a theological argument informally known as the Kairos Document. See Kairos Theologians, *A Challenge to the Church: A Theological Comment on the Political Crisis in South Africa* (Grand Rapids: Eerdman, 1986). The document was originally published in South Africa in 1985. At publication, the document had over 150 signatories representing 22 different Christian bodies in South Africa. The moral power displayed through the process was replicated

both in subsequent movements in South Africa and also in other countries, most notably in the occupied territories in Palestine.

8 See Emmanuel Katongole, *The Sacrifice of Africa: A Political Theology of Africa* (Grand Rapids: Eerdmans, 2010); Mercy Amba Oduyoye, *Beads and Strands: Reflections of an African Woman on Christianity in Africa* (Maryknoll, NY: Orbis, 2002); Emmanuel Katongole, et. al. *African Theology Today* (Eugene, OR: Wipf and Stock, 2017).

9 See Thomas O'Brien, "The Nixon-Cronin Speeches: A Cold War Theology," in *Toronto Journal of Theology* 10, no. 1 (1994): 53–80; Dianne Kirby, et. al. *Religion and the Cold War* (New York: Palgrave MacMillan, 2003); Mahmood Mamdani, *Good Muslim, Bad Muslim: America, the Cold War, and the Roots of Terror* (New York: Pantheon, 2004).

10 See Andrew Preston, "Peripheral Visions: American mainline Protestants and the global Cold War," in *Cold War History* 13, no. 1 (2013): 109–130; Max Guderzo and Bruna Bagnato, eds. *The Globalization of the Cold War: Diplomacy and local confrontation, 1975–1985* (New York: Routledge, 2010).

11 For an excellent summary of this kind of theological thinking, see Elaine Graham, Heather Walton, and Frances Ward, *Theological Reflection: Methods* (London: SCM Press, 2005). See especially, Chapter 6: Theology-In-Action: Praxis. Also, see Gustavo Gutierrez, *A Theology of Liberation* (Maryknoll, NY: Orbis, 1973).

12 Ada Maria Isasi-Diaz, *Mujerista Theology: A Theology for the Twenty-first Century* (Maryknoll, NY: Orbis, 1996). Andrew Sung Park, *The Wounded Heart of God: The Asian Concept of Han and the Christian Doctrine of Sin* (Nashville: Abingdon, 1993). Also, see Graham, Walton, and Ward, chapter 7.

13 For information on the the Circle, see their website at www.thecirclecawt.com

14 See Elizabeth A. Clarke and Herbert Richardson, eds. *Women and Religion: An Original Sourcebook in Christian Thought* (New York: Harper One, 1996); Beverly Wildung Harrison and Elizabeth Bounds, *Justice in the Making: Feminist Social Ethics* (Louisville: Westminster John Knox, 2004); Elizabeth A. Johnson, *She Who Is: The Mystery of God in Feminist Theological Discourse* (New York: Crossroad Publishing, 1992); Rosemary Radford Ruether, *Sexism and God-Talk: Toward a Feminist Theology* (Boston: Beacon Press, 1993 edition); Sheila Briggs and Mary McClintock Fulkerson, eds. *The Oxford Handbook of Feminist Theology* (New York: Oxford University Press, 2014 edition).

15 James Cone, *A Black Theology of Liberation* (Maryknoll: Orbis, 2011 edition); Dwight Hopkins, *Being Hunan: Race, Culture, and Religion* (Philadelphia: Fortress Press, 2005); Dwight Hopkins and Edward Antonio, eds. *The Cambridge Companion to Black Theology* (New York: Cambridge University Press, 2014).

16 Delores Williams and Katie Cannon, *Sisters in the Wilderness: The Challenge of Womanist God-Talk* (Maryknoll: Orbis, 2013); Monica Coleman, *Making a Way Out of No Way: A Womanist Theology* (Philadelphia: Fortress, 2008); Jacquelyn Grant, *White Woman's Christ and Black Woman's Jesus: Feminist Christology and Womanist Response* (Atlanta: Scholars Press, 1989); Katie Cannon and Emilie Townes, eds. *Womanist Theological Ethics: A Reader* (Louisville: Westminster John Knox, 2011).

17 Marcella Althaus-Reid, *The Queer God* (New York: Routledge, 2003); Daniel Boisvert and Jay Johnson, eds. *Queer Religion (2 Volumes)* (New York: Praeger, 2011); Mark Jordan, *The Invention of Sodomy in Christian Theology* (Chicago: University of Chicago Press, 1997); John Boswell, *Christianity, Social Tolerance and Homosexuality* (Chicago: University of Chicago Press, 2015 edition).

18 James T. Patterson, "The Moynihan Future," in *The New York Times*, May 29, 2010, p. A25.

19 Daniel P. Moynihan, *The Negro Family: The Case for National Action* (Washington, DC: U.S. Department of Labor, 1965), 29.

20 Benjamin F. Payton, "New Trends in Civil Rights," in *Christianity and Crisis* 25, no. 21 (1965): 270.

21 Benjamin Payton, "Black Power: A Statement by the National Committee of Negro Churchmen," in *The New York Times* July 31, 1966, p. 143.

22 James F. Findlay, *Church People in the Struggle: The National Council of Churches and The Black Freedom Movement, 1950–1970* (New York: Oxford University Press, 1993), 186.

23 Bill Clinton, "Remarks by the President in Apology for Study Done in Tuskegee," (speech, Washington, DC, May 16, 1996); Online: https://clintonwhitehouse4.archives.gov/textonly/New/Remarks/Fri/19970516-898.html, accessed March 6, 2018.

24 Presidential Commission for the Study of Bioethical Issues, *"Ethically Impossible" STD Research in Guatemala from 1946 to 1948* (Washington, DC: Presidential Commission for the Study of Bioethical Issues, 2011), 76.
25 Cornell West, *Opening Plenary to the American Public Health Association* (speech, Denver, CO, November 7, 2010), www.youtube.com/watch?v=kjZydhfUxqs, accessed March 13, 2018.
26 This term is recounted by Paula Treichler as commonplace in New York City in the early days of the epidemic. See Paula Treichler, *How to Have Theory in an Epidemic* (Durham, NC: Duke University Press, 2004), 27.
27 *Executive Committee of the World Council of Churches, AIDS and the Churches* (Geneva: WCC Publications, 1986), www.oikoumene.org/en/resources/documents/executive-committee/1986/aids-and-the-churches, accessed March 7, 2018.
28 See www.oikoumene.org/en/what-we-do/ehaia for further information.
29 For more information on the Ecumenical Advocacy Alliance, see www.oikoumene.org/en/what-we-do/eaa
30 www.oikoumene.org/en/resources/documents/wcc-programmes/diakonia/ehaia/documents-on-hiv-and-aids
31 For further information on INERELA+, visit the organization's website at Online: http://inerela.org
32 Halfdan Mahler, "Annual Report of the Director General on the Work of WHO in 1976,"in *Official Records of the World Health Organization, No. 241: Thirtieth World Health Assembly, Part II*, pp. 51–56 (Geneva: World Health Organization, 1977), 53–54, Online: http://apps.who.int/iris/bitstream/10665/86037/1/Official_record241_eng.pdf, accessed March 13, 2018.
33 A list of participants is available on the WHO website at Online: http://apps.who.int/iris/bitstream/10665/69504/1/ICPHC_ALA_78.10_eng.pdf, accessed February 27, 2018. There are debates regarding what exactly constitutes a faith-based organization. The Aga Khan Foundation identifies itself as faith-inspired but explicitly notes that its programs are determined by health and social science research and not religious doctrines.
34 World Health Organization, "Declaration of Alma-Ata," in *Report of International Conference on Primary Health Care* (Geneva: World Health Organization, 1978), 2–6.
35 See Robert W. Cox, "Ideologies and the New International Economic Order: Reflections on Some Recent Literature," in *International Organization* 33, no. 2 (1979): 257–302. For a discussion on the effects of these economic policies on public health written around the time in which they were being debated, see Oscar Gish, "The Relation of the New International Economic Order on Health," in *Journal of Public Health Policy* 4, no. 2 (1983): 207–221.
36 "Primary Health Care Comes Full Circle," in *Bulletin of the World Health Organization* 86, no. 10: 748.
37 Halfdan Mahler, *Address to the 61st World Health Assembly* (speech, Geneva, May 20, 2008), www.who.int/mediacentre/events/2008/wha61/hafdan_mahler_speech/en/, accessed March 17, 2018.

References

Althaus-Reid, Marcella. *The Queer God*. New York: Routledge, 2003.

Boisvert, Daniel and Jay Johnson, eds. *Queer Religion (2 Volumes)*. New York: Praeger, 2011.

Boswell, John. *Christianity, Social Tolerance and Homosexuality*. Chicago: University of Chicago Press, 2015 edition.

Briggs, Sheila and Mary McClintock Fulkerson, eds. *The Oxford Handbook of Feminist Theology*. New York: Oxford University Press, 2014 edition.

Cannon, Katie and Emilie Townes, eds. *Womanist Theological Ethics: A Reader*. Louisville: Westminster John Knox, 2011.

Christian Medical Commission. "The Beginning—Tübingen I, 1964." In *Contact*, Special Series, no. 2 (1979):1–6.

Clarke, Elizabeth A. and Herbert Richardson, eds. *Women and Religion: An Original Sourcebook in Christian Thought*. New York: Harper One, 1996.

Clinton, Bill. "Remarks by the President in Apology for Study Done in Tuskegee." Speech, Washington, DC, May 16, 1996. https://clintonwhitehouse4.archives.gov/textonly/New/Remarks/Fri/19970516-898.html. Accessed March 6, 2018.

Coleman, Monica. *Making a Way Out of No Way: A Womanist Theology*. Philadelphia: Fortress, 2008.

Cone, James. *A Black Theology of Liberation*. Maryknoll: Orbis, 2011 edition.

Cox, Robert W. "Ideologies and the New International Economic Order: Reflections on Some Recent Literature." *International Organization* 33, no. 2 (1979): 257–302.

Executive Committee of the World Council of Churches. "AIDS and the Churches." Geneva: WCC Publications, 1986. www.oikoumene.org/en/resources/documents/executive-committee/1986/aids-and-the-churches. Accessed March 7, 2018.

Findlay, James F. *Church People in the Struggle: The National Council of Churches and The Black Freedom Movement, 1950–1970*. New York: Oxford University Press, 1993.

Gish, Oscar. "The Relation of the New International Economic Order on Health." *Journal of Public Health Policy* 4, no. 2 (1983): 207–221.

Graham, Elaine, Heather Walton, and Frances Ward. *Theological Reflection: Methods*. London: SCM Press, 2005.

Grant, Jacquelyn. *White Woman's Christ and Black Woman's Jesus: Feminist Christology and Womanist Response*. Atlanta: Scholars Press, 1989.

Grundmann, Christopher H. "The Legacy of Tubingen I." In *Christian Responses to Health and Development: Symposium at the German Institute for Medical Mission (DIFAEM), pp. 12–25*, 18–19. Tübingen: DIFAEM, 2014.

Guderzo, Max, and Bruna Bagnato, eds. *The Globalization of the Cold War: Diplomacy and local confrontation, 1975–1985*. New York: Routledge, 2010.

Gustavo, Gutierrez. *A Theology of Liberation*. Maryknoll, NY: Orbis, 1973.

Harrison, Beverly Wildung and Elizabeth Bounds. *Justice in the Making: Feminist Social Ethics*. Louisville: Westminster John Knox, 2004.

Hopkins, Dwight. *Being Human: Race, Culture, and Religion*. Philadelphia: Fortress Press, 2005.

Hopkins, Dwight and Edward Antonio, eds. *The Cambridge Companion to Black Theology*. New York: Cambridge University Press, 2014.

Isasi-Diaz, Ada Maria. *Mujerista Theology: A Theology for the Twenty-first Century*. Maryknoll, NY: Orbis, 1996.

Johnson, Elizabeth A. *She Who Is: The Mystery of God in Feminist Theological Discourse*. New York: Crossroad Publishing, 1992.

Jordan, Mark. *The Invention of Sodomy in Christian Theology*. Chicago: University of Chicago Press, 1997.

Kairos, Theologians. *A Challenge to the Church: A Theological Comment on the Political Crisis in South Africa*. Grand Rapids: Eerdman, 1986.

Katongole, Emmanuel. *The Sacrifice of Africa: A Political Theology of Africa*. Grand Rapids: Eerdmans, 2010.

Katongole, Emmanuel, et al. *African Theology Today*. Eugene, OR: Wipf and Stock, 2017.

King, William McGuire. "The Emergence of Social Gospel Radicalism: The Methodist Case." *Church History* 50, no. 4 (Dec., 1981): 436–449.

Kirby, Dianne, et al. *Religion and the Cold War*. New York: Palgrave MacMillan, 2003.

Litsios, Socrates. "The Christian Medical Commission and the Development of the World Health Organizations Primary Health Care Approach." *American Journal of Public Health* 94, no. 11 (2004): 1884–1893.

Mahler, Halfdan. "Annual Report of the Director General on the Work of WHO in 1976." In *Official Records of the World Health Organization, No. 241: Thirtieth World Health Assembly, Part II*, 51–56. Geneva: World Health Organization, 1977. http://apps.who.int/iris/bitstream/10665/86037/1/Official_record241_eng.pdf. Accessed March 13, 2018.

Mahler, Halfdan. "Address to the 61st World Health Assembly." Speech, Geneva, May 20, 2008. www.who.int/mediacentre/events/2008/wha61/hafdan_mahler_speech/en/. Accessed March 17, 2018.

Mamdani, Mahmood. *Good Muslim, Bad Muslim: America, the Cold War, and the Roots of Terror*. New York: Pantheon, 2004.

McGilvray, James. *The Quest for Health and Wholeness*. Tübingen, The German Institute for Medical Mission, 1981.

Moynihan, Daniel P. *The Negro Family: The Case for National Action*. Washington, DC: U.S. Department of Labor, 1965.

O'Brien, Thomas. "The Nixon-Cronin Speeches: A Cold War Theology." *Toronto Journal of Theology* 10, no. 1 (1994): 53–80.

Oduyoye, Mercy Amba. *Beads and Strands: Reflections of an African Woman on Christianity in Africa*. Maryknoll, NY: Orbis, 2002.

Park, Andrew Sung. *The Wounded Heart of God: The Asian Concept of Han and the Christian Doctrine of Sin*. Nashville: Abingdon, 1993.

Patterson, James T. "The Moynihan Future." *The New York Times*, May 29, 2010, p. A25.

Payton, Benjamin. "Black Power: A Statement by the National Committee of Negro Churchmen." *The New York Times*, July 31, 1966, p. 143.

Payton, Benjamin F. "New Trends in Civil Rights." *Christianity and Crisis* 25, no. 21, 1965: 268–271.

Phiri, Isabel Apawo. "The Healing Ministry of the Churches Today." In *Christian Responses to Health and Development: Symposium at the German Institute for Medical Mission (DIFAEM)*, 5–11. Tübingen: DIFAEM, 2014.

Presidential Commission for the Study of Bioethical Issues. *"Ethically Impossible" STD Research in Guatemala from 1946 to 1948*. Washington, DC: Presidential Commission for the Study of Bioethical Issues, 2011.

Preston, Andrew. "Peripheral Visions: American mainline Protestants and the Global Cold War." *Cold War History* 13, no. 1 (2013): 109–130.

"Primary Health Care Comes Full Circle." *Bulletin of the World Health Organization* 86, no. 10: 747–748.

Ruether, Rosemary Radford. *Sexism and God-Talk: Toward a Feminist Theology*. Boston: Beacon Press, 1993 edition.

Treichler, Paula. *How to Have Theory in an Epidemic*. Durham, NC: Duke University Press, 2004.

West, Cornell. "Opening Plenary to the American Public Health Association." Speech, Denver, CO, November 7, 2010. www.youtube.com/watch?v=kjZydhfUxqs. Accessed March 13, 2018.

Williams, Delores and Katie Cannon. *Sisters in the Wilderness: The Challenge of Womanist God-Talk*. Maryknoll: Orbis, 2013.

World Health Organization. "Declaration of Alma-Ata." In *Report of International Conference on Primary Health Care*, 2–6. Geneva: World Health Organization, 1978.

6 American Protestantism in the Cold War

The influence of liberal Protestantism on global health and development initiatives within the United Nations and the WCC was strong and long-lasting. This in-depth Christianization as a manifestation of a secularized Social Gospel designed to transfer the empire of the world from the United States to other nations was not, however, the only ways in which American Protestantism intersected with national and international politics in the years after World War II. As that war ended, another one began and it would last for the next 45 years: the Cold War. Once again, religion influenced America's perceptions of this global issue; more importantly it influenced America's foreign policy of containment in contexts and through programs far removed from the United Nations and the WCC.

American Protestantism and the Cold War

One of the most influential religious leaders in this context was the Protestant theologian Reinhold Niebuhr. An early champion of the Social Gospel, he eventually came to develop a sharp critique of the movement for its failure to deal with issues of power and politics. And so, while Niebuhr shared Rauschenbusch's critiques of capitalism and actually complained about Roosevelt's New Deal policies because they did not go nearly far enough,[1] he believed that the Social Gospel champions were naïve to believe that nations could be molded into utopias in which global war would cease, arguing that

> the use of force to restrain evil was defensible, even required, on the grounds of Christian ethics, whether in the struggle for justice on the part of suffering workers in the domestic arena or in the fight against aggression in the international. Christianity is not solely a religion of love. It is more properly a religion of judgment and justice that requires difficult, even tragic, choices, in which one must sometimes engage in evil for the sake of doing good.[2]

In 1932, Niebuhr wrote *Moral Man and Immoral Society*. In it, he laid out the basic contours that he would develop in the coming decades: human beings are imperfect and although we are in the throes of sin, we can weigh our options and choose good. Therefore, we have moral responsibility even as we face the tragedy that sometimes our choices will be immoral because of our imperfections. When this dynamic moves beyond the individual to the societal, the stakes are exponentially higher: we have the moral responsibility to fashion more just societies but we will inevitably choose wrongly, especially at the corporate level. Christians can neither optimistically assume that society is perfectible—a swipe at the political naiveté of the Social Gospel—nor retreat into a bunker when concrete threats emerge—a swipe at isolationism. Rather we have to weigh our options in an imperfect world marred by sin in which political power is afoot. We get our hands messy and we cannot rely on the nation to craft a perfect society in that complex, imperfect, messy world; in fact, when we recognize political power being misused, we have an obligation to employ power to respond.

Niebuhr emphasized strikingly different aspects of Christian theology from his Social Gospel peers and the theological viewpoints he developed became influential with political leaders who were determining the nation's foreign policy response to the emergence of the Soviet Union. George Kennan, U.S. Ambassador to the Soviet Union in the early 1950s, was instrumental in crafting the U.S. policy of containment. Speaking for these foreign policy leaders Kennan called Niebuhr "the father of us all."[3]

In a 1947 article in *Foreign Affairs*, the journal of the Council on Foreign Relations, Kennan laid out the based argument that would eventually underwrite America's containment policy. He framed the relationship between the United States and the Soviet Union in providential terms:

> The thoughtful observer of Russian-American relations will find no cause for complaint in the Kremlin's challenge to American society. He will experience a certain gratitude to a Providence which, by providing the American people with this implacable challenge, has made their entire security as a nation dependent on their pulling themselves together and accepting its responsibilities of moral and political leadership that history plainly intended them to bear.[4]

In short, Kennan reflected the same perspectives first articulated 200 years earlier regarding America's providential role as a moral light to the world. This was a perspective Niebuhr also put forth in arguing that America's leaders "had a providential destiny to provide political leadership to the world, despite their political and moral flaws, because the United States was politically, morally, and spiritually superior to its new rival."[5] In the eighteenth century, Protestant leaders preached a vision of America's providential role in saving the world by embodying God's kingdom on earth; in the twentieth century, the nation's government leaders reiterated that message of American responsibility to fulfill its responsibilities reflecting the moral and political leadership bestowed to the nation by Providence.

Just as Protestant Christianity was a force in rallying Americans in support of the United Nations and in articulating a holistic community-based model of primary health care, it was also an instrument in America's Cold War effort, a factor in how the United States fought the Soviet Union. At the same time, however, liberal Protestantism had lost its hegemony. Since the nation's founding, Protestantism had served as the *de facto* voice of America's religious ideals; in the face of growing religious diversity America's religious leaders worked to articulate a rhetoric of American exceptionalism rooted in a generalized, common religiosity. In the 1940s and 1950s, the nation's political leaders—especially Presidents Truman and Eisenhower—developed the language of America's civil religion.[6]

Harry S. Truman, civil religion, and the Cold War

In 1946, less than a year after the end of World War II, Truman sent a letter to the General Assembly of the Presbyterian Church of the USA:

> Religion and democracy in this country . . . have mutually strengthened each other . . . Here, as perhaps nowhere else in the world, the fundamental unity of Christianity and freedom has been demonstrated. Religion alone has the answer for humanity's twentieth century cry of despair, 'What must I do to be saved?' In this time of grave anxiety the voice of science unites with the voice of religion to affirm that the words of Jesus, "Do good to them that hate you," are not only the words of Christian idealism but also the command of democratic realism.[7]

For Truman, religion offered a bulwark against malevolent forces in times "of grave anxiety." It united with other sources of knowledge—"the voice of science"—to re-enforce the commandment handed down by Christ himself. That commandment to return hatred with good, Truman claimed, informed not only the Christian idealism of the Social Gospel, the World Council of Churches, or the United Nations; it was also required when fashioning America's foreign policy—a policy that came to be known as democratic realism—in the Cold War stalemate with the Soviet Union that was coming into focus. Truman often demonstrated an appreciation for various religious traditions, expressing the belief that each of them represented different paths to common universal truths. In an entry in his personal diary, Truman referenced the Golden Rule:

> The combined thought and action of the whole people of any race, creed, or nationality will always point in the Right Direction: "As ye would that others

> should do unto you do ye also unto them." Confucius, Buddha, Christ, and all moralists come to the same conclusion.

What he could not abide was the atheism he saw as central to the Soviet Union's communist system. In the same diary entry, he wrote: "Honest Communism, as set out in the 'Acts of the Apostles,' would work. But Russian Godless Pervert Systems won't work."[8]

He did not, however, envision some unification of religions and American interests only on the pages of his diary. In fact, Truman attempted an inter-religious initiative to promote American ideals and condemn communism. Again, for Truman, such an alliance was possible because he minimized theological differences and emphasized political and moral commonalities based on his interpretation of moral principles such as the Golden Rule. Truman believed that such moral principles represented a powerful response to the dangers of Soviet communism. The President's representatives met with a number of European religious leaders, including the Pope, the Archbishop of Canterbury, the Lutheran Bishop of Berlin, the Catholic Bishop of London, and the Papal Nuncio in Paris to present the American proposal

> that if people of all religious faiths would, in the present world crisis, unite upon a universal two-point declaration embodying the spirit of belief in God and belief in human liberty, to which mankind would dedicate itself, it might help temporarily and be effective permanently in bringing people to a better basis of understanding in the interest of world peace.[9]

Truman soon discovered that religious leaders were skeptical of such a plan. In a meeting between invited Protestant clergy and governmental officials in October 1947, the religious leaders attending raised objections to the proposal for minimizing differences across religions and for making ecumenical global Christian bodies instruments of the U.S. government:

> The whole operation is based on a very naive view of the relationship of the churches and the world religions . . . The WCC is not an association to stop communism, nor an effort to block atheism as such . . . I wish our President could be disabused of the idea that there is some moral unity in Mohammedanism, in Judaism and Christianity that could be associated structurally or in an informal way to stop the on-rush of communism or of atheism.[10]

Protestants, then, were not enthusiastic supporters of Truman's plan. The next year, it was dealt another blow when the patriarchs of the Orthodox Churches in both Greece and Russia declined a meeting to discuss their support. But then, in July 1949, Truman received unexpected good news for his American civil religion.

Pope Pius XII issued a decree in which any Catholic who was a member of supporter of the Community Party or who printed, publicized, read, or wrote materials in support of communist positions or practices would be subject to excommunication.[11] Truman's envoy to the Pope (the United States did not establish formal diplomatic relations with the Vatican until 1984) informed the President that the Vatican would "most warmly welcome collaboration with Protestants in the common fight of religious persons against the communist atheists" and assured the President that "a Vatican official described these events as a 'great turning point' in Catholic-Protestant relations, on the same scale as the 1520 papal bull denouncing the Protestant reformers, with the crucial difference that [there was an opportunity now for] unity instead of division."[12]

With clear indications from Vatican officials that the Roman Catholic church was open to a stronger relationship with Protestant leaders, Truman pushed ahead. His administration began to make plans for a global inter-religious gathering in Washington, DC. In personal communications to his staff, Truman wrote:

> My prayer will ever be that we may again achieve in the quest for a true peace something of the spirit of tolerance, understanding, and good will which enabled Catholics, Protestants, Jews and men and women of all faiths whether Mohammedans, Buddhists or Hindus to submerge their religious differences during the fighting war . . . against the totalitarian enemies whom we together faced in that challenging ordeal. I think we should aim to enlist the active interest and support of all nations in a new quest for peace, based on unity of moral values and on common belief in one God who is Lord of Lords, and King of Kings.[13]

For two years, the administration met with resistance from religious leaders who were concerned that the traditions they represented would be co-opted by the politics of the day. Under Truman's persuasion, however, both Pope Pius XIII and Episcopal bishop Henry Knox Sherrill who had just been appointed as President of the National Council of Churches, began to warm to the idea of a global gathering in which a statement would be produced.

And then the entire enterprise fell apart—not over political concerns but over theological disputes. Pope Pius had proclaimed the Bodily Assumption of the Virgin Mary as an infallible teaching of the church. Protestants were incensed and argued that their nascent fears of a Roman Catholicism mired in strident dogmatism had come true. The Archbishops of York and Canterbury issued a joint statement from the Anglican communion complaining that

> The Church of England does not and cannot hold this doctrine to be a necessary part of the Catholic faith, belief in which may be required of members of the church . . . We profoundly regret that the Roman Catholic Church has

> chosen by this act to increase dogmatic differences in Christendom and has thereby gravely injured the growth of understanding between Christians.[14]

Truman's long-held hope for a strong statement from the world's religious leaders against communism fell apart; ironically, the effort failed in the end not because of the leaders' misgivings about having their traditions subsumed under a statement of general moral principles in the services of the political interests of the United States. Rather, Truman's effort to craft a creed for his civil religion failed because of internal theological differences between Protestants and Catholics—differences he had long minimized in order to privilege a common voice in support of Western democratic ideals.

Truman, however, was still eager to deploy religion as a weapon in his fight against Soviet communism in the Cold War. In 1951, he created a top-secret initiative called the Psychological Strategy Board. In a classified memo to the U.S. Central Intelligence Agency, the State Department, the National Security Council, and the Defense Department, the Board wrote:

> The potentialities of religion as an instrument for combating Communism are universally tremendous. Religion is an established basic force which calls forth men's strongest emotions. Because of the immoral and un-Christian nature of Communism and its avowed opposition to and persecution of religions, most of the world's principal religious organizations are already allied with the cause of the free nations. Our over-all objective in seeking the use of religion as a cold war instrumentality should by the furtherance of world spiritual health; for the Communist threat could not exist in a spiritually healthy world.[15]

The memo urged the government to use its resources and relationships to

> publicize at every opportunity the threat communism posed to religious belief, that religious leaders continue to provide policy guidance to the State Department in this area, and that the State Department "encourage churches, their leaders, and their members to oppose Communist doctrine and practices." And so the last year of the Truman Administration saw the beginnings of a systematic effort by the U.S. government to employ religion as an ideological weapon in the effort to contain Soviet communism.[16]

Truman was clearly a missionary for the Cold War gospel of American civil religion. He was determined to spread that message across the globe through as many religious and governmental channels as he could create.

His worries about the communist menace, however, did not end with the Soviet Union and its satellite states in eastern Europe. With the fall of Chiang Kai-shek as leader of the Nationalist Party in 1949, China joined the USSR as an emerging communist power. The United States had had a long-time missionary presence in China; in time that presence ironically helped catalyze the revolution, according to John Fairbank, a well-known Chinese historian. Fairbank argued that missionary efforts not only to preach the gospel but to attend to social, economic, health, and educational needs (the focus of global health and development) served to awaken millions of Chinese to the inequities they faced. While missionary efforts revealed the tremendous gaps that existed in Chinese societies they were nonetheless insufficient to bridge those gaps:

> The missionaries came as spiritual reformers, but soon found that material improvements were equally necessary, and in the end helped to foment the great revolution. Yet as foreigners, they could take no part in it, much less bring it to finish. Instead, it finished them.[17]

We like Ike: President Eisenhower's distinctly American Christianity

The week following his inauguration as President of the United States, Dwight Eisenhower and his wife Mamie met in private with the Session—the lay leadership—of the National Presbyterian Church on Connecticut Avenue in Washington, DC. The Session asked Eisenhower to testify to his faith in Jesus Christ, which he did. Following this meeting, the Session and the ministers of the congregation conducted a small, private baptism service for Eisenhower followed by the liturgy of confirmation of the faith; Mrs. Eisenhower, who had been baptized and then confirmed into the Presbyterian church in her childhood, watched. That following Sunday, February 1, 1953, the Eisenhowers were introduced as new members during the 9 AM service and then joined the congregation in the ritual of communion.[18] Eisenhower is the only U.S. President to be baptized while in office. A new convert to Christianity, he also seemed to be a good spokesperson to the nation. His two terms as President were marked by increased church attendance among American citizens and an unabashed religiosity in American culture.

However, the depth of Eisenhower's faith was always a matter of debate. Why, some wondered, hadn't Eisenhower been baptized earlier and why did he so often choose to play a round of golf on Sunday mornings rather than attend church?[19] Matthew Neely, a Democratic Senator from West Virginia, named Eisenhower "a publican" for his frequent, public showings of religiosity that had no grounding in a deeper faith. However, Eisenhower also had his defenders, especially in regard to Neely's charge, with other politicians, members of the general public, and religious leaders (both Protestant and Catholic) calling Neely out of bounds.[20] At a meeting with his cabinet early in his administration, Eisenhower forgot to open with a time of silent prayer, a practice he had instituted. The cabinet secretary slipped the President a note to remind him. Seeing the note, Eisenhower famously replied, "Goddammit, we forgot the silent prayer."[21]

By and large, it seems, America supported Eisenhower's public displays of religious devotion and ignored contrary evidence that such displays were only surface deep. The news of Eisenhower's expletive regarding his memory lapse over prayer was met more with amusement than outrage. But there was one exhortation to prayer that became politically important for Eisenhower in his shepherding of America's civil religion and his effort to enlist that religion in the Cold War fight.

A key event in that enlistment occurred at the Second World Assembly of the World Council of Churches, held in Evanston, Illinois, in 1954. The background of the Cold War impacted the event and a pamphlet published by the WCC for the assembly raised pointed critiques of both communism and liberal democracy. The report said that communism offers

> an exciting world of false hope for the down-trodden. But communism must fall because of its denial of God, the Marxist belief that proletarian man can act as his own Messiah for a new age, and the fact that actual Marxist behavior does not bear out the theory that strife and self-seeking can be abolished under communism.

Democratic humanism was also criticized, but for different reasons: "a disregard or denial of God's sovereignty over the world, and failure to recognize the imperfect, precarious and transient character of all human achievements."[22]

President Eisenhower spoke at the World Assembly less than a year into his administration. President Eisenhower had carried on Truman's efforts to enlist religious leaders as spokespersons against communism. The WCC equivocation of communism and democracy undoubtedly bothered him. Nonetheless, Eisenhower didn't address the issue; he didn't utter one word about communism or democracy. But he did manage to shift the conversation with his words:

> Let me speak then, for a moment, not as this Nation's Chief Executive, whose days are largely devoted to the efforts of Government to secure peace, but as a private citizen, a single member of one of the constituent bodies of this Council of Churches. . . .
>
> Today—now—the campaign for a just and lasting peace desperately needs the lifting and transforming power that comes from men and women the world over, responding to their highest allegiance and to their best motives.
>
> Now, how can we help strike this spark of dedication in receptive hearts around the earth? I believe that you, members of this convocation, spiritual leaders of a great world organization, together with your brethren of other faiths, can lead the way.

> The goal should be nothing short of inviting every single person, in every single country in the world, who believes in the power of a Supreme Being, to join in a mighty, simultaneous, intense act of faith. That act of faith might take the form of a personal prayer, delivered simultaneously and fervently, by hundreds upon hundreds of millions who have the devotion, wisdom, and stamina to work unceasingly for a just and lasting peace. If this mass dedication launched an unending campaign for peace, supported constantly by prayer, I am certain wondrous results would ensue.
>
> First, and at the very least, there would be a reminder to each of us that the cause of peace needs God. We would come to know also that responsibility for peace or conflict rests in some degree with each of us. Each would be heartened and strengthened by the certainty of close comradeships in faith and purpose. Thus there would be set in motion a great and growing force that could unify men in peace as a common peril unifies them in war.[23]

Without ever mentioning Soviet Russia or communism, Eisenhower changed the debate. Who could object to a worldwide prayer for peace? Certainly not the Protestant theologians from around the world who crafted the controversial pamphlet.

With his call for prayer, Eisenhower set up an implied link between the desire for peace and the American side in the Cold War while also isolating the Soviet Union by never once invoking the Cold War. Only the most fervent communist-atheist could object to a "prayer for peace," so in one fell homiletical swoop Eisenhower attempted to isolate the Kremlin and bring the "spiritual" peoples of the world into the American camp. Various media lauded the President for his words. The American newsweekly *Time Magazine* said that the speech "captured perfectly the fundamental series of relationships between God, order, freedom, and peace."[24] *Life* Magazine was far more effusive. Without ever mentioning the critique of democracy, the magazine published an editorial on the World Assembly declaring that "Christianity itself is the living and revolutionary force which alone can halt Communism, and which alone can save the world from its greatest peril—destruction by the H-bomb." The editorial then referenced the President's speech specifically:

> The President suggested worldwide prayer as a "mighty, simultaneous, intense act of faith." The council agreed; it set aside next Jan. 18 to 25 as a week of universal prayer. Let us all mark it down; let us pray. And let us pray many times in the interim . . . The best role for all God-fearing men is not only to pray but to bring constant, continuing pressure upon the President to hunt new ways to solve this paramount issue. And he must seek the world's prayers, time and again, in the hope that enough faith *can* move even the Soviet mountain.[25]

Eisenhower had succeeded in recruiting Christians and anyone else who "believes in the power of a Supreme Being" worldwide to become not only "prayer warriors" but also "Cold Warriors" without ever uttering a word about Cold War conflict.

Eisenhower shocked observers and American allies in 1956 by aligning the United States against the activities of England, France, and Israel during the Suez crisis. This decision created political capital for Eisenhower among Muslim-majority nations and when the President and Mrs. Eisenhower visited the opening of the Islamic Center in Washington, DC, in 1957, newspapers across the Middle East highlighted the story of their visit with a photo of them taking off their shoes to enter into the mosque. Leading mullahs in Iran called the White House, expressing their appreciation. The administration used this goodwill to build stronger alliances with strategic nations in the Middle East as an effort to thwart any Soviet gains in the region.[26]

In all of these events, Eisenhower attempted to find common ground among various religious traditions—that common ground being American patriotism in the midst of the Cold War. He was the first President who had to negotiate the loss of liberal Protestant hegemony in the culture, the concurrent first steps of evangelicalism to enter into the political space, the social changes occurring from the entry of millions of American-born children of Eastern and Southern European Catholic immigrants into adulthood, and growing non-Christian religious communities. The civil religion first articulated by Truman and then later expanded by Eisenhower at the height of American religiosity was a new phenomenon but it had a long pedigree that could be traced across American Protestantism for almost 300 years. Will Herberg, an influential American sociologist, claimed that "from the very beginning the American Way of Life was shaped by the contours of American Protestantism; it may, indeed, be best understood as a kind of secularized Puritanism. Having identified itself so closely with American culture, American Protestantism now found itself needing to evolve in response to changes within that culture—not only a growing pluralism at home, but the sinister foe abroad that threatened all religion."[27]

Sober calculations: public health during the Cold War

On August 9, 1945, at 10 PM in the evening, President Harry S. Truman addressed the nation via radio. The title of his address references his return from the Potsdam Conference, in which the Allied Powers were negotiating the terms of peace with the European Axis Powers. The speech, however, is remembered for the President's discussion of atomic weapons. Three days earlier, the United States had dropped the world's first atomic bomb used in war on the city of Hiroshima and in his address, President Truman affirmed the nation's choice to use the bomb and promised it would do so again until Japan no longer maintained the capacity to wage war:

> Having found the bomb we have used it. We have used it against those who attacked us without warning at Pearl Harbor, against those who have starved

> and beaten and executed American prisoners of war, against those who have abandoned all pretense of obeying international laws of warfare. We have used it in order to shorten the agony of war, in order to save the lives of thousands and thousands of young Americans. We shall continue to use it until we completely destroy Japan's power to make war. Only a Japanese surrender will stop us.[28]

Truman made no reference to the bombing of Nagasaki, which, astoundingly, had happened that very day. Near the end of his address, he remarked,

> It is an awful responsibility which has come to us. We thank God that it has come to us, instead of to our enemies. And we pray that He may guide us to use it in His ways and for His purposes.

Truman's senior staff indicated that the thought of the bombing of Nagasaki was "too horrible" for the President. Perhaps. Indeed, the bombing was different from that which had occurred in Hiroshima three days earlier. It resulted in a far higher number of civilian deaths because the bomb missed its target and detonated over a mostly civilian district. Military plans to warn the citizens of Nagasaki and of other target cities to evacuate their cities failed because only a small number of senior military officials knew of the second attack. As a result, the American planes carrying leaflets warning of a possible future attack dropped their warnings over Nagasaki the day *after* the bomb was detonated. Truman had expressly removed himself from the decision chain for the bombs up until this point, leaving the decision to the nation's military leaders. After Nagasaki, he changed that policy; no more bombs would be dropped without his express authorization.[29] There would be no need for any more bombs. Six days after the bombing of Nagasaki, Japan surrendered and the Second World War came to an end. The Nuclear Age, however, had begun.

In his study of the public health response to the threat of nuclear war, anthropologist Joseph Masco has argued that the threat of the atomic bomb inverted our assessments of health and security, demanding that we define these terms in relation to death.[30] With exhortations of national security, the Cold War response to the nuclear threat in the United States instilled in its citizens the realization that total destruction was a constant possibility and then provided mechanisms for us to accept it as good citizens.

In the first years of the Cold War, America's civil defense efforts focused on instilling an emotional adjustment within the American public to equip them to deal with this omnipresent, constant threat. The government carried out a dizzying number of projects with this purpose of turning terror at the threat of nuclear war into an anxiety that could be managed. The public health goal was not an absence of anxiety but a self-discipline predicated on the normalization of the threat facing the citizens.

Since the emergence of modern nations, one of the key functions of government was the regulation of health and the provision of security. The Cold War, says Masco, required an entirely new model of security because the government could not guarantee survivability of the threat for the general public. The government's security focus minimized the threat of nuclear war and focused on the political, cultural, and economic containment of the "Soviet menace."This required an unprecedented escalation of nation's defense budget, including significant funds channeled into social and economic development in strategic locations. It also required recruiting America's citizens as Cold Warriors. But how could public health officials address the terror inherent in the atomic bomb while also avoiding apathy? "The solution," Masco said, "was a new kind of project, one pursued with help from social scientists and the advertising industry, to teach citizens a specific kind of cognitive and emotional attitude toward the bomb."[31] Through civil defense films and literature, community meetings, bomb drills, and educational programs, the nation's public health services taught Americans to fear the bomb but not to be terrorized by its threats—to "transform 'nuclear terror,' which was interpreted by officials as a paralyzing emotion, into 'nuclear fear,' an emotional state that would allow citizens to function in a time of crisis."[32] Reading the public health documents of the era and the narratives of officials working on the public health response at the time, Masco's analysis is insightful.

Dr. George Moore recounted his efforts as part of the U.S. Public Health Service (USPHS) to coordinate medical care plans for five Midwestern states in the event of a nuclear attack. Moore's efforts under the auspices of the USPHS focused on emergency preparedness and response:

> We attempted to persuade each individual, in addition to groups and government agencies, that he or she had a measure of responsibility to the collective whole. Public as well as private preparedness could mean the difference between national survival and extinction.[33]

That responsibility was shared by the government's public health officials as

> we endeavored to allay panic and assure people that everything possible was being done to provide them with a plan for survival. Our objective was to teach people how to respond to a disaster and to use the tools we offered. The most important element was to help people survive the initial attack so that they could begin to help themselves and others recover for the long term.[34]

In his conclusions, Moore explicitly mirrors Masco's analysis in writing that

> the threat of war, particularly one as encompassing as a nuclear war, can render individuals and communities vulnerable and helpless. Our plans actively

> involved every member of the community to some degree, equipping them with a plan of responsibility that each member could carry out. Even if they did not feel more secure, they felt as though they were contributing to a greater cause and doing everything possible to help themselves and others to survive.[35]

In 1953, the director of the Federal Civil Defense Administration (FCDA) wrote a piece entitled "Panic: The Ultimate Weapon?"

> What will you do if one day an atomic bomb blasts your town? Will you take calm emergency action—or will you dash screaming into the ruined streets a victim of your own terror? In a war, the whole country's survival could depend on your reaction to disaster . . . because mass panic may be far more devastating than the bomb itself. We must not let uncontrolled fear conquer us in an emergency—and the time to start taking precautions is right now. . . .
>
> Ninety percent of all emergency measures after an atomic blast will depend on the prevention of panic among the survivors in the first 90 seconds. Like the A-bomb, panic is fissionable. It can produce a chain reaction more deeply destructive than any explosive known. If there is an ultimate weapon, it may well be mass panic—not the A-bomb. . . .
>
> Panic can be fought and conquered if a free people are informed, prepared, have useful activity, good leadership and sound faith. No nation can win which allows itself to be stampeded. None can be defeated which has a clear, unbreakable will to resist.[36]

In 1946, six months after the United States had dropped the bombs, the Federal Council of Churches (FCC) released a document entitled *Atomic Warfare and the Christian Faith*. It demonstrates just how fully the violence, destruction, and death of the second world war had changed the theological tone. There is no remnant of the Social Gospel rhetoric of progress or the possibility of building a worldly utopia. Rather, two themes are prominent.

First, the document demonstrates a deep cynicism toward technology and a skepticism that human beings have the wisdom to responsibly and ethically deploy scientific knowledge for the good:

> Our latest epochal triumph of science and technology may prove to be our last. The scientists who know most about the nature of atomic energy have been the first to declare themselves frightened men. With admirable restraint, but with impressive urgency, they have sought to awaken both military leaders and civilians to the alarming realities which as scientists they see more clearly than laymen who lack their special knowledge . . . The basis of any hope for the redemption of mankind simply through progress in the sciences and

> technology, always an unsound hope, has been permanently wrecked by the latest achievement in that very progress.[37]

Second, the report communicates remorse and sorrow and states that there was no justifiable use of the bombs:

> We would like to begin with an act of contrition. As American Christians, we are deeply penitent for the irresponsible use made of the atomic bomb. We are agreed that, whatever be one's judgment of the ethics of war in principle, the surprise bombing of Hiroshima and Nagasaki are morally indefensible . . . Both bombings . . . must be judged to have been unnecessary for winning the war. Japan's strategic position was already hopeless, and it was virtually certain that she had not developed atomic weapons of her own. Even though use of the new weapon last August may well have shortened the war, the moral cost was too high.[38]

Critical words, no doubt. However, in August 1949, the Soviet Union successfully detonated a nuclear bomb and the rhetoric changed. In 1950, just weeks before its dissolution and reconstitution as the National Council of Churches, the FCC released a second document on the threat of nuclear war. Entitled *The Christian Conscience and Weapons of Mass Destruction*, the document had different focuses from the document four years earlier. The document now argued that the United States now had a moral responsibility not to disarm but to manage nuclear weapons judiciously:

> The only possible justification for war is that it offers a possibility of achieving a moral result, however imperfect, to prevent an overwhelming moral evil and to offer a new opportunity for men to live in freedom and decency and in just and merciful relationships . . . As long as the existing situation holds, for the United States to abandon its atomic weapons, or to give the impression that they would not be used, would leave the non-communist world with totally inadequate defense. For Christians to advocate such a policy would be for them to share responsibility for the world-wide tyranny that might result. We believe that American military strength, which must include atomic weapons as long as any other nation may possess them, is an essential factor for the possibility of preventing both world war and tyranny.[39]

As a second point, the document articulated a strategy to move the world away from the brink of nuclear war—concerted, global efforts in social and economic development:

> Fatalism and defeatism which assumes the inevitability of war with world Communism deflects us from the very strategy which offers us the hope of any real victory: namely, the building up of the economic and social and moral health

> of the areas in our world not already under complete Communist domination. For Communism is more than the tyranny and imperial ambitions of the Soviet rulers. It is also a political religion, whose promise of a universal, classless society, tragically perverted though they have been, still carry a dynamic appeal to those oppressed by harsh and unjust conditions. To overcome such conditions requires positive non-military measures.[40]

Systematic and sustained foreign aid from the United States government took root in the Truman and Eisenhower administrations, evolving from nascent programs in the Philippines after the Spanish-American War and the State Department's Institute for Inter-American Affairs during World War II. This shift also reflected the eclipse of denominationally funded foreign missions' initiatives as such governmental programs came to the fore. Truman's inauguration speech spelled out the "Point Four" origins of foreign aid and laid the groundwork for the creation of the U.S. Agency for International Development, or USAID. Foreign assistance initiatives revealed both American efforts to support social and economic development in poorer countries and the nation's own strategic priorities, using aid dollars as an instrument to further its own interests. The Cold War context meant that foreign assistance initiatives were impacted by Soviet initiatives and responses. This interplay was readily evident even in the first large-scale assistance initiative after the end of World War II—the Marshall Plan.

The destruction in Europe caused by the War reflected a humanitarian crisis. The human, social, and economic costs of the war weighed heavily on the continent and its governments in the aftermath or the war and the United States government allocated a total of $13 billion toward the Marshall Plan, the popular name for an initiative known as the European Recovery Program in reference to U.S. Secretary of State George Marshall, who oversaw the recovery efforts. The plan had widespread support from Protestant religious leaders. As the U.S. Congress was holding hearings on the plan and considering funding levels, the Federal Council of Churches published a pamphlet entitled *Churches Support of the European Recovery Program*. The pamphlet stated, "As Christians, we support the European recovery program in the conviction that it can be one of history's most momentous affirmation of faith in the curative power of freedom and in the creative capacity of free men. The ways and means of that program will, of necessity, be largely economic and political. The motives and objectives behind it should be essentially moral and spiritual."[41]

Pope Pius XII offered his enthusiastic support of the plan, with caveats. In his book, *Religion and American Foreign Policy 1945–1960*, William Inboden, a former senior staff of the National Security Council and now a professor of public policy, details the interchange between the Pope and President Truman. In July 1948, Pope Pius sent a letter to Truman, which Inboden describes as follows:

> No doubt reinforcing Truman's own belief in a providential role for America, the Pope declaimed that "on the foreign policy of the United States of America

> chiefly hinges the issue of the fateful struggle between what remains of a free world and God-less totalitarianism." The Pope singled out the "Marshall Plan as a particularly notable, and noble, initiative. To succeed, however, it must follow certain principles. European recovery must be seen as an end in its own right and not just a crass tool used to contain the Soviets. The American people must support their government and embrace European recovery as a worthy goal. Finally, it would not be sufficient to focus on just one European country. All of Europe must be revived, and a spirit of cooperation and independence must be established and "guaranteed by some international authority." Fearful of resurgent German hegemony as well as Soviet designs on the continent, the Pope threw his firm support behind a European mutual security regime. Political and economic reform alone would not do. "Any program of assistance will fail of its purpose unless it takes into account the imperative need for men to return to God."[42]

Truman was thrilled at the Vatican's strong support, and in his reply to Pope Pius, he framed the Marshall Plan not in political terms, but in explicitly biblical ones:

> The primary purpose of the Marshall plan was and is to bind up the wounds of war, to feed the hungry, to give shelter to the homeless. Through labor and industry, with the blessing of God, these sorely stricken nations shall again become masters of their own destiny.[43]

The Marshall Plan was unquestionably a catalyst in the economic recovery of Europe after the war; it was also one of the catalysts of the Cold War.

In the aftermath of the war, the Soviet Union initially supported talks in the United Nations to carry out rebuilding efforts in Europe. Soviet involvement in those talks soon broke down, however, and Andrei Vyshinsky, the Soviet Ambassador to the UN, spoke from the floor of the General Assembly to denounce the plan:

> The United States government has moved towards a direct renunciation of the principles of international collaboration and concerted action by the great powers and towards attempts to impose its will on other independent states, while at the same time obviously using the economic resources distributed as relief to individual needy nations as an instrument of political pressure . . . This policy conflicts sharply with the principle expressed by the General Assembly in its resolution of 11 December 1946, which declares that relief supplies to other countries "should . . . at no time be used as a political weapon."
>
> As is now clear, the Marshall Plan constitutes in essence merely a variant of the Truman Doctrine adapted to the conditions of postwar Europe. In bringing forward this plan, the United States government apparently counted on

> the cooperation of governments of the United Kingdom and France to confront the European countries in need of relief with the necessity of renouncing their inalienable right to dispose of their economic resources and to plan their national economy in their own way. The United States also counted on making all these countries directly dependent on the interests of American monopolies, which are striving to avert the approaching depression by an accelerated export of commodities and capital to Europe. . . .
>
> It is becoming more and more evident to everyone that the implementation of the Marshall Plan will mean placing European countries under the economic and political control of the United States and direct interference by the latter in the internal affairs of those countries.
>
> Moreover, this plan is an attempt to split Europe into two camps and, with the help of the United Kingdom and France, to complete the formation of a bloc of several European countries hostile to the interests of the democratic countries of Eastern Europe and most particularly to the interests of the Soviet Union.
>
> An important feature of this plan is the attempt to confront the countries of Eastern Europe with a bloc of Western European states including Western Germany. The intention is to make use of Western Germany and German heavy industry (the Ruhr) as one of the most important economic bases for American expansion in Europe, in disregard of the national interests of the countries which suffered from German aggression.[44]

In reality, the use of aid as implemented in the Marshall Plan specifically and in America's foreign policy more generally contained motivations that reflected Truman's letter to the Pope and the UN speech by a Soviet critic. In 1951, speaking with a group of Methodist leaders at the White House, Truman stated that

> the United States Government has no ambitions as a colonial power or as an exploiter of people or other races. Our only ambition is to see that the people in the world have the things that are necessary to make life worthwhile, and that they have and live by the moral code in which we believe. That is the fundamental principle of the foreign policy of the United States.[45]

America realized that it faced structural challenges when using aid to further its own strategic interests. In 1959, the historian Norman Graebner laid out those challenges in a briefing document that included both a policy analysis and an American condescension to "the backward regions" who received American foreign aid. He argued that "foreign aid comprises a response to a challenge, and that challenge lies partially in the widespread poverty of Asia and Africa, and partially in the American concept of the cold war in the non-European world." Graebner argued that the Soviet Union had ramped up its foreign aid initiatives beginning in 1956, and he laid out two advantages the Soviets possessed in this arena. First, because the Soviet Union had no alliance with the colonizing nations in these regions they could feign personal disinterest and frame their aid as evidence of Soviet compassion (Graebner doesn't address the fact that the negative perceptions of colonialism were not the fault of those colonized or merely the result of Soviet propaganda, but the effect of the colonizers implementing a social-political system of domination):

> Russia has advantages over the West in penetrating the underdeveloped nations through policies of trade and aid. Having no tradition of 'colonialism' in the regions of South and Southeast Asia or the Middle East, the Kremlin can make its pretense of disinterestedness appear exceedingly plausible. The Soviet leaders, moreover, need not stress self-interest to gain support at home for expensive foreign aid policies.

Second, communism offered a more feasible route for economic development than capitalism, which required an initial critical mass of capital that these nations simply did not possess:

> Every national economy requires a capital fund large enough to sustain its own economic expansion. Countries with primitive economic levels have no local surplus of capital for expansion of the economy. The U.S.S.R. has shown that a nation can build its economy through controlled production and consumption rather than awaiting the slow accumulation of capital through the profits of private enterprise.[46]

And so, Truman's policy of containment—a policy so defining of his foreign policy agenda that it came to be known as the Truman Doctrine—was not directed only at Soviet Russia; it had clear implications for developing nations because of America's strategy of using development dollars as a strategic instrument in carrying out the Truman Doctrine. The government intervened in the affairs of these nations through the leverage of these dollars with one eye toward social and economic development and another toward cultural Americanization. These programs reflected the "progressive imperialism" of Teddy Roosevelt and Woodrow Wilson employed a half century earlier. Such interventions were not only humanitarian; they were political, leveraging economic and military power to influence the makeup of some nations' governments or even to install new regimes in nations not supportive of American interests:

> Foreign aid, much of which was military, was used as carrot and stick. Acceptance of the structure of capitalism, including market access and investor export of profits, was usually a condition of aid. Receipt of foreign aid was also coupled to the recipient country's political restructuring, which required that

> Communists and left-wing Socialists be excluded from government. Securing consent for these fundamental requirements typically included seducing local elites through the offer of aid (and bribes). If these didn't succeed at elevating American- backed groups, the United States would help local clients repress opponents by force or by helping facilitate coups d'état.[47]

For Truman and Eisenhower, religion was an important instrument in furthering their political agendas. However, both men also expressed religious motivations that were not simple political calculations as evidenced by their personal writing. Their administrations welcomed the support of religious leaders even though that such support was often conditional. Foreign aid policies reflected this dynamic. In a 1957 meeting with Eisenhower and the Secretary of State John Foster Dulles, U.S. representatives from the CCIA of the World Council of Churches urged the administration to emphasize economic development assistance over military aid, arguing "that our government's programs of technical and economic aid can increasingly be planned and administered in relation primarily not to political and military considerations but to economic and social needs and opportunities." Their advocacy had an effect, at least rhetorically. When Dulles went to Congress to push for increased foreign aid funding later that year, he distinguished between developmental and military aid and argued for economic development on the grounds of American interests; he also argued for it on the grounds of the universal mutuality of humankind under the moral law, and the need to extend freedom. For their part, the CCIA representatives had also stepped away from a Social Gospel optimism that Niebuhr had characterized as naïve and demonstrated a realism so characteristic of the period: "While the proposal as a whole falls far short of an adequate program, it represents I suspect about as much as can be achieved at the present time."[48]

In the early Cold War years, Truman and Eisenhower employed American Protestantism in the rhetoric of an American civil religion, sometimes with the support of the movement's leaders. Even as the infrastructure for global health and development initiatives was being developed during these decades through the structures of the United Nations agencies and through funding of the United States government (among others), the strategies of Cold War politics were also assessing religion's capacity to further America's interests in fighting "the Soviet menace" by influencing popular opinion. In these efforts, the nation's political leaders as well as its religious leaders were eager to ensure that the transfer of Empire would not proceed only to the communist world.

Notes

1 Robert B. Horwitz, "The Revival of Reinhold Niebuhr: A Foreign Policy Fable," in *Public Culture* 28, no. 1 (2015): 120.
2 Ibid., p. 114.

3 George Rice, *Reinhold Niebuhr and His Circle of Influence* (New York: Cambridge University Press, 2013), 174.
4 George Kennan, "The Sources of Soviet Conduct," in *Foreign Affairs* 25, no. 4 (1947): 582. The article had been written as a private report to the Secretary of Defense James Forrestal and was initially published anonymously.
5 S.R. Thompson and James K. Wellman, "The Social Gospel Legacy in U.S. Foreign Policy," in *Interdisciplinary Journal of Research on Religion* 7, no. 6 (2011): 33
6 The American historian Walter McDougall defines civil religion in this way: "A civil religion is a set of beliefs and attitudes that explain the meaning and purpose of an given political society in terms of its relationship to a transcendent, spiritual reality, that are held by the people generally of that society, and that are expressed in public rituals, myths, and symbols." See Walter A. McDougall, *The Tragedy of U.S. Foreign Policy: How America's Civil Religion Betrayed the National Interest* (New Haven, CT: Yale University Press, 2016), 30.
7 William Inboden, *Religion and American Foreign Policy, 1945–1960: The Soul of Containment* (New York: Cambridge University Press, 2008), 110.
8 Ibid., p. 108. The capitalization in the quote is from the citation. "The Acts of the Apostles" is a book in the New Testament that represents a sacred text for Christians. Passages in the book (especially in chapters 2, 4, and 5) have been interpreted to reflect a socio-economic model more in keeping with twentieth-century communism than free market capitalism.
9 Ibid., p. 124.
10 Ibid., p. 138.
11 Peter C. Kent, *The Lonely Cold War of Pope Pius XII: The Roman Catholic Church and the Division of Europe, 1943–1950* (Montreal: McGill-Queen's University Press, 2002), 242–253.
12 Inboden, p. 143.
13 Ibid., p. 145
14 "Anglicans Assail New Rome Dogma: Archbishops of York and Canterbury Say Pope's Action Will Undermine Christian Unity," *The New York Times*, August 18, 1950, p. 17.
15 Jonathan P. Herzog, *The Spiritual-Industrial Complex: America's Religious Battle Against Communism in the Early Cold War* (New York: Oxford University Press, 2011), 126.
16 Inboden, p. 118.
17 John Fairbanks, *The Missionary Enterprise in China and America* (Cambridge, MA: Harvard University Press, 1974), 2.
18 "Faith Staked Down,"Time 61, no 6 (1953): 20.
19 Andrew Preston, *Sword of the Spirit, Shield of Faith: Religion in American War and Diplomacy* (New York: Alfred A. Knopf, 2012), 442.
20 Gary Scott Smith, *Faith and the Presidency: From George Washington to George W. Bush* (New York: Oxford University Press, 2006), 226.
21 Herbert S. Parmet, Eisenhower and the American Crusades (New York: Macmillan, 1972), 176.
22 "Churches Assail Democracy Flaws; Report by World Council Unit Also Declares Communism False and Sure of Doom," *The New York Times*, June 15, 1954, p. 27.
23 Dwight Eisenhower, *Address at the Second Assembly of the World Council of Churches* (speech, Evanston, IL, August 19, 1954). The American Presidency Project, www.presidency.ucsb.edu/ws/?pid=9991, accessed February 24, 2018.
24 "Under God,"Time 64, no. 9 (1954): 9.
25 "Editorial: A Path to Peace Through Prayer," in *Life Magazine* 37, no. 11 (1954): 48.
26 Ibid., pp. 291–292.
27 Will Herberg, *Protestant, Catholic, Jew: An Essay in American Religious Sociology* (New York: Doubleday and Company, 1955), 81.
28 Harry S. Truman, *Radio Report to the American People on the Potsdam Conference* (speech, Washington, DC, August 9, 1945). The American Presidency Project, www.presidency.ucsb.edu/ws/?pid=12165, accessed February 25, 2018.
29 Alex Wellerstein, "Nagasaki: The Last Bomb," in *The New Yorker*, online edition, August 7, 2015. www.newyorker.com/tech/elements/nagasaki-the-last-bomb, accessed February 25, 2018.
30 Joseph Masco, "Atomic Health, or How the Bomb Altered American Notions of Death," in *Against Health: How Health Became the New Morality*, eds. Jonathan M. Metzl and Anna Kirkland, pp. 133–154 (New York: New York University Press, 2010).

31 Ibid., p. 143.
32 Ibid., p. 180.
33 George Moore, "Threats to Our Nations, 1957–1959: A Public Health Retrospective," in *Public Health Reports* 124, no. 2 (2009): 324.
34 Ibid.
35 Ibid., p. 326.
36 Val Peterson, "Panic: The Ultimate Weapon?" *Colliers Weekly*, August 21, 1953, pp. 100, 109.
37 *Commission on the Relation of the Church to the War in Light of the Christian Faith, Atomic Warfare and the Christian Faith: Report of the Commission on the Relation of the Church to the War in the Light of the Christian Faith* (New York: Federal Council of Churches, 1946), 4, 7.
38 Ibid., p. 10.
39 Department of International Justice and Goodwill, *The Christian Conscience and Weapons of Mass Destruction* (New York: Federal Council of Churches, 1950), 11, 14.
40 Ibid., pp. 16–17.
41 *Churches Support of the European Recovery Program* (New York: Federal Council of Churches of the United States, 1948). The contents of the pamphlet were published in their entirety in the February 12, 1948 meetings of the House Committee on Foreign Affairs. Those minutes are available online through the archives of the Marshall Foundation. See Online: http://marshallfoundation.org/library/wp-content/uploads/sites/16/2014/05/Section_14i.pdf. The pamphlet text is on the first three pages of the scanned document, which are pages 1181–1183 of the original report.
42 Inboden, p. 137.
43 Inboden, pp. 112, 137.
44 Michael Holm, *The Marshall Plan: A New Deal for Europe* (New York: Routledge, 2017), 149–150.
45 Harry S. Truman, "Remarks to a Gathering of Methodist Ministers," in *Public Papers of the Presidents of the United States*, Harry S. Truman, *Containing the Public Messages, Speeches, and Statements of the President, January 1, 1951-December 31, 1951* (Washington, DC: U.S. Government Printing Office, 1965), 141.
46 Norman Graebner, "Foreign Aid: A Strategy in the Cold War," in *Increasing Understand of Public Problems and Policies: 1959 edition* (Oak Brook, IL: Farm Foundation, 1959), 20–21.
47 Horwitz, p. 123.
48 Inboden, pp. 247–248.

References

"Anglicans Assail New Rome Dogma: Archbishops of York and Canterbury Say Pope's Action Will Undermine Christian Unity." *The New York Times*, August 18, 1950, p. 17.

Churches Support of the European Recovery Program. New York: Federal Council of Churches of the United States, 1948.

"Churches Assail Democracy Flaws; Report by World Council Unit Also Declares Communism False and Sure of Doom," *The New York Times*, June 15, 1954, p. 27.

Commission on the Relation of the Church to the War in Light of the Christian Faith. *Atomic Warfare and the Christian Faith: Report of the Commission on the Relation of the Church to the War in the Light of the Christian Faith*. New York: Federal Council of Churches, 1946.

Department of International Justice and Goodwill. *The Christian Conscience and Weapons of Mass Destruction*. New York: Federal Council of Churches, 1950.

"Editorial: A Path to Peace Through Prayer." *Life Magazine* 37, no. 11 (1954): 48.

Eisenhower, Dwight. "Address at the Second Assembly of the World Council of Churches." Speech, Evanston, IL, August 19, 1954. The American Presidency Project. www.presidency.ucsb.edu/ws/?pid=9991. Accessed February 24, 2018.

Fairbanks, John. *The Missionary Enterprise in China and America*. Cambridge, MA: Harvard University Press, 1974.

"Faith Staked Down." *Time* 61, no. 6 (1953): 20.

Graebner, Norman. "Foreign Aid: A Strategy in the Cold War." *Increasing Understand of Public Problems and Policies: 1959 edition*. Oak Brook, IL: Farm Foundation, 1959.

Herberg, Will. *Protestant, Catholic, Jew: An Essay in American Religious Sociology*. New York: Doubleday and Company, 1955.

Herzog, Jonathan P. *The Spiritual-Industrial Complex: America's Religious Battle Against Communism in the Early Cold War*. New York: Oxford University Press, 2011, 126.

Holm, Michael. *The Marshall Plan: A New Deal for Europe*. New York: Routledge, 2017.

Horwitz, Robert B. "The Revival of Reinhold Niebuhr: A Foreign Policy Fable." *Public Culture* 28, no. 1 (2015): 113–138.

Inboden, William. *Religion and American Foreign Policy, 1945–1960: The Soul of Containment*. New York: Cambridge University Press, 2008.

Kennan, George. "The Sources of Soviet Conduct." *Foreign Affairs* 25, no. 4 (1947): 566–582.

Kent, Peter C. *The Lonely Cold War of Pope Pius XII: The Roman Catholic Church and the Division of Europe, 1943–1950*. Montreal: McGill-Queen's University Press, 2002.

Masco, Joseph. "Atomic Health, or How the Bomb Altered American Notions of Death." In *Against Health: How Health Became the New Morality*, eds. Jonathan M. Metzl and Anna Kirkland, 133–154. New York: New York University Press, 2010.

McDougall, Walter A. *The Tragedy of U.S. Foreign Policy: How America's Civil Religion Betrayed the National Interest*. New Haven, CT: Yale University Press, 2016.

Moore, George. "Threats to Our Nations, 1957–1959: A Public Health Retrospective." *Public Health Reports* 124, no. 2 (2009): 323–327.

Parmet, Herbert S. *Eisenhower and the American Crusades*. New York: Macmillan, 1972.

Peterson, Val. Panic: The Ultimate Weapon? *Colliers Weekly*, August 21, 1953, pp. 99–109.

Preston, Andrew. *Sword of the Spirit, Shield of Faith: Religion in American War and Diplomacy*. New York: Alfred A. Knopf, 2012.

Rice, George. *Reinhold Niebuhr and His Circle of Influence*. New York: Cambridge University Press, 2013.

Smith, Gary Scott. *Faith and the Presidency: From George Washington to George W. Bush*. New York: Oxford University Press, 2006.

Thompson, S. R. and James K. Wellman. "The Social Gospel Legacy in U.S. Foreign Policy." *Interdisciplinary Journal of Research on Religion* 7, article 6 (2011): 41.

Truman, Harry S. "Remarks to a Gathering of Methodist Ministers." In *Public Papers of the Presidents of the United States, Harry S. Truman: Containing the Public Messages, Speeches, and Statements of the President, January 1, 1951-December 31, 1951*, 141–142. Washington, DC: U.S. Government Printing Office, 1965.

Truman, Harry S. "Radio Report to the American People on the Potsdam Conference." Speech, Washington, DC, August 9, 1945. The American Presidency Project. www.presidency.ucsb.edu/ws/?pid=12165. Accessed February 25, 2018.

"Under God." *Time* 64, no. 9 (1954): 9.

Wellerstein, Alex. "Nagasaki: The Last Bomb." *The New Yorker*. Online edition, August 7, 2015. www.newyorker.com/tech/elements/nagasaki-the-last-bomb. Accessed February 25, 2018.

7 No longer on the mainline

Other Christianities, other religions, and no religion

The resurgent interest in religion displayed in the fields of global health and international development over the last 15 years has largely been informed by the legacy of global Christian Protestantism embodied in both religious and secular organizations such as the Christian Medical Commission of the World Council of Churches and the World Health Organization—the world of Alma-Ata. Likewise, the religious, political, and cultural world that birthed those institutions can't be completely understood apart from the earlier iterations of eighteenth- and nineteenth-century liberal Protestantism. This, however, is not the world we inhabit in 2018. Liberal Protestantism is no longer the epicenter of political and cultural power and the United Nations is met with suspicion in the United States today as often as support. The social history of American Protestantism and its influences on America's global health and development policies and programs has been the subject of this book. However, such a social history remains incomplete without also examining the different religious landscapes in America at this point in time. This chapter examines the influences of American evangelicalism, Roman Catholicism, and the religious "nones" (people who express religious or spiritual beliefs but are not part of any religious tradition) in the social and political landscapes of America today.

Changes in American Christianity in the latter half of the twentieth century

Demographic shifts among Protestants in America

In 1961, when the 87th American Congress convened, all 532 members formally announced an affiliation with a religious tradition. Christians overwhelmingly dominated, with 95% of the members indicating membership in a Christian tradition. In 2015, when the 113th Congress convened, only one of the 535 members declared that they had no religious affiliation and 92% of members still called themselves Christian. Despite the tremendous cultural changes in the United States and the rest of the world in the 54 years between the 87th and the 113th Congress, the religious affiliations had not changed significantly (see Table 7.1).

What had changed was the representation of different Christian traditions. There were 92 fewer Protestant Christians in the 113th Congress, a decrease of 23%. The number of Roman Catholics skyrocketed from 100 to 164. Reflecting the growth in the number of Christian congregations that labeled themselves nondenominational, there were 62 nondenominational or unspecified Christian in 2015 where there had only been 28 in 1961 (see Table 7.2).

Table 7.1 Religious affiliation of members of the United States Congress, 1961–1962 and 2015–2016.

	87th Congress (both House and Senate) 1961–1962	*%*	*113th Congress (both House and Senate) 2015–2016*	*%*
Christian (all types)	505	94.9	491	91.8
Jewish	12	2.2	28	5.2
Buddhist	0	0	2	.4
Muslim	0	0	2	.4
Hindu	0	0	1	.2
Other	10	1.9	1	.2
Unaffiliated	0	0	1	.2
Refused	5	1	9	1.6
	532		535	

Source: "Faith on the Hill." The Pew Research Center on Religion and American Life, 2015.. www.pewforum.org/2015/01/05/faith-on-the-hill/.

Table 7.2 Denominational affiliation of Christians in the United States Congress, 1961–1962 and 2015–2016.

	87th Congress (both House and Senate) 1961–1962	*113th Congress (both House and Senate) 2015–2016*	*% change*
PROTESTANT	398	306	–23.1%
Baptist	62	79	
Methodist	*97*	*45*	*–53.6%*
Presbyterian	*73*	*36*	*–50.7%*
Episcopal	*66*	*41*	*–37.9%*
Lutheran	*21*	*27*	*28.6%*
Nondenominational	0	4	
Restorationist	18	3	
Holiness	0	1	
Congregationalist	*27*	*4*	*–85.2%*
Adventist	0	2	
Christian Scientist	4	2	
Pentecostal	0	3	
Reformed	1	1	
Friends	2	0	
Anabaptist	2	0	
Pietist	2	0	
Unspecified	23	58	
CATHOLIC	100	164	64.0%
MORMON	7	16	128.6%
ORTHO. CHRISTIAN	0	5	

Note: The rows shaded gray represent mainline Protestant denominations. Source: Faith on the Hill.

All of the decrease among Protestant Christians can be attributed to the sharp drop in numbers of mainline Protestants. Their loss of 133 members more than offset gains made among evangelical Protestant members. Collectively, there were 47% fewer mainline Protestant members of Congress in 2015 than in 1961; among the entire membership, mainline Protestants made up 54% of Congress in 1961 and only 29% in 2015 (see Table 7.3).

This shift in the Congress is just as pronounced in the general public. An analysis of the seven largest mainline Protestant congregations—the United Methodist Church; the Episcopal Church; the Presbyterian Church (USA); the Evangelical Lutheran Church in America; the American Baptist Churches in the USA; the United Churches of Christ; and the Christian Church, Disciples of Christ reveals striking losses in membership when compared to three of the largest evangelical or Pentecostal Protestant denominations—the Southern Baptist Convention, the Lutheran Church—Missouri Synod, and the Assemblies of God. From 1952 to 2010, the total number of members in those seven denominations decreased by about 1.3 million people, or about 6%, even as the nation's population more than doubled; as a result, the percentage of the nation's population represented by these denominations shrank by more than half, from over 15% to about 7%. The three evangelical Protestant denominations fared far better, doubling their membership between 1952 and 1980 to over 25 million members. From 1980 to 2010, the total membership among these denominations has basically reflected the population growth of the United States and they represent 8% of the nation's population. Some of the other large Christian traditions are growing with the Mormon church experience a seven-fold growth over the last 60 years and Roman Catholic has remained steady—19.7% of the population in 1952 and 19.1% in 2010 (see Table 7.4).

Mainline Protestantism still retains a great deal of cultural power and the influence of its various institutions remains impressive. Nonetheless, it is no longer the *de facto* religious voice of American culture. This does not mean that the mainline churches are in their death throes, despite prognoses by some conservative evangelicals such as Albert Mohler, President of Southern Baptist Theological Seminary and one of the leaders of the Southern Baptist Convention, who says of the tradition: "Once the vital content of the Christian faith is removed, denied, or marginalized, all that remains is a vaguely Christian spirituality and an agenda of social activism."[1] Such proclamations fail to account for membership drops in theologically conservative

Table 7.3 Members of the United States Congress who are members of mainline Protestant denominations, 1961–1962 and 2015–2016.

	87th Congress (both House and Senate) 1961–1962	*113th Congress (both House and Senate) 2015–2016*	*%change*
# of Mainline Protestants	286	153	–46.5%
% of total members	53.8%	28.6%	

Source: Pew Research Center on Religion and Public Life. Source Faith on the Hill.

Table 7.4 Select denominational representation among American Christians, 1952–2010.

	1952		*1980*		*1990*		*2000*		*2010*	
	Members	*% U.S. Pop*	*Members*	*% U.S. Pop*	*Members*	*% U.S. Pop*	*Members*	*% U.S. Pop*	*Members*	*% U.S. Pop*
Evangelical										
SBC	8,121,069	5.4%	16,281,692	7.2%	18,940,682	7.6%	19,881,467	7.1%	19,896,279	6.4%
AoG	459,256	0.3%	1,612,655	0.7%	2,161,610	0.9%	2,561,998	0.9%	2,944,887	1.0%
Miss. Synod	1,835,605	1.2%	2,622,847	1.2%	2,603,725	1.0%	2,521,062	0.9%	2,270,921	0.7%
TOTAL	*10,415,930*	*6.9%*	*20,517,194*	*9.1%*	*23,706,017*	*9.5%*	*24,964,527*	*8.9%*	*25,112,087*	*8.1%*
Mainline										
UMC	8,790,025	5.8%	11,552,111	5.1%	11,091,032	4.5%	10,350,629	3.7%	9,860,653	3.2%
PCUSA	3,415,794*	2.3%	4,012,835	1.8%	3,553,335	1.4%	3,141,566	1.1%	2,451,980	0.8%
ELCA	3,281,982	2.2%	5,379,943	2.4%	5,226,798	2.1%	5,113,418	1.8%	4,181,219	1.4%
ECA	2,544,320	1.7%	2,823,399	1.2%	2,445,286	1.0%	2,314,756	0.8%	1,951,907	0.6%
ABCUSA	1,528,846	1.0%	1,922,467	0.9%	1,873,731	0.8%	1,767,462	0.6%	1,560,572	0.5%
UCC	2,013,935**	1.3%	2,096,014	0.9%	1,993,459	0.8%	1,698,918	0.6%	1,284,296	0.4%
Disciples	1,836,104	1.2%	1,212,977	0.5%	1,037,757	0.4%	1,017,784	0.4%	785,776	0.3%
TOTAL	23,411,006	15.5%	28,999,746	12.8%	27,221,398	10.9%	25,404,533	9.0%	22,076,403	7.2%
Latter-Day Saints	*845,689*	*0.6%*	*2,684,744*	*1.2%*	*3,540,820*	*1.4%*	*4,224,026*	*1.5%*	*6,144,582*	*2.0%*
Catholic	*29,688,058*	*19.7%*	*47,502,152*	*21.0%*	*53,385,998*	*21.5%*	*62,035,042*	*22.0%*	*58,963,835*	*19.1%*
Other/None	*89,618,660*	*59.5%*	*131,583,579*	*58.2%*	*146,082,438*	*58.7%*	*169,908,521*	*60.4%*	*200,629,850*	*65.0%*
US Population	**150,697,361**		**225,907,472**		**248,709,873**		**281,423,231**		**308,745,538**	

Source: U.S. Religious Census, www.usreligioncensus.org/compare.php

denominations, including Mohler's own Southern Baptist denomination in the last few years. Rather, liberal Protestantism is now part of a much more diverse religious landscape (both within Christianity and in a nation with other non-Christian traditions), and it carries out quite different roles in America today. These roles also influence global health and development policies and practices, albeit in different ways from the liberal Protestantism of a century ago.

American evangelicalism emboldened

The 1950s saw the first stirrings of a social shift in America's religious landscape that would have implications in the coming decades: the re-emergence of American evangelicalism in American politics. After the fundamentalist-modernist controversies of the 1920s, the rhetoric of personal salvation and soul conversion was not often invoked in mainline Protestantism or in the government's civil religious discourse. While evangelicalism was not identical to fundamentalism, both movements were critical of what they perceived to be the dangers of liberalism in the church and both had largely chosen an approach of separatism after the controversies of the 1920s subsided. During Eisenhower's administrations, evangelicals began more direct, active political engagement.

The American Council of Churches, a conservative evangelical parallel body to mainline Protestantism's National Council of Churches, had urged the President not to speak at the Second World Assembly in Evanston, equating the World Council of Churches—especially some theologians and religious leaders from Eastern European nations—with communist sympathizers.[2] Although Eisenhower did not heed their request, evangelicals were optimistic about the direction of the country in the Eisenhower years. Church membership among Americans in 1956 topped 100 million with 61% of the citizens a member of a church body, up from 57% in 1950 and 49% in 1940.[3]

The National Association of Evangelicals (NAE) had formed in 1943, but a decade later, its leadership began to organize politically. In 1954, the body's leadership—including Billy Graham and Harold Ockenga, the President of Fuller Theological Seminary—strategized ways in which the group could counter the social and political power they saw growing among Roman Catholics. In a memo on the issue, the leadership of the NAE warned that: "the only way to head off the Roman Catholic menace to our nation is by using the same legal tactics they do, and that is 'legal infiltration' of the various branches of our government."[4] Working together, Graham, his father-in-law, Nelson Bell, and Ockenga launched a new magazine they called *Christianity Today* geared toward American evangelicals by offering an alternative to the liberal *Christian Century*. They sought funding for the magazine from Howard Pew, President of the Sun Oil Company (Sunoco); convinced of the need of the magazine to combat the dangers he saw in secularism and liberalism, Pew bankrolled the magazine and remained involved in its management until his death in 1971.

Christianity Today provided evangelicals with a new platform for advocacy and political involvement. The National Council of Churches, World Council of Churches, and the United Nations, and America's foreign aid policy were frequent objects of the magazines sharp criticisms.[5] In short, the magazine was focused on rebutting the entire framework of late nineteenth- and early twentieth-century Protestantism embodied in the Social Gospel.

At the time, Eisenhower seemed largely unaware of the growing political power of American evangelicalism. Most in his administration equated their stricter theology with a more narrow constituency, confusing it with fundamentalism. When the NAE contacted Eisenhower in 1953, asking him to articulate a clear public stand of his belief in God and to sign their Declaration of Freedom, Eisenhower and his senior staff were unsure how to respond. White House staff contacted the Library of Congress asking them to research the NAE specifically and evangelicalism more broadly. In the end, the administration was ambivalent about this expression of Christianity they had never experienced: while the body was fairly large, representing about ten million Christians, it excluded "modern" Christians. While the body was patriotic and unabashedly anti-Communist it was also "a highly determined group of Biblical Fundamentalists,"[6] according the Library of Congress response.

The precipitous drop in membership among mainline Protestant denominations from the 1950s into the 2000s has offered evidence to Evangelicals and to other conservative Americans whatever their religious affiliations that liberalism and Christianity are not compatible. These critics of liberal Protestantism criticize the tradition as theologically shallow and a rehash of secular liberalism with a dash of non-dogmatic Jesus thrown in:

> This decline is the latest chapter in a story dating to the 1960s. The trends unleashed in that era—not only the sexual revolution, but also consumerism and materialism, multiculturalism and relativism—threw all of American Christianity into crisis, and ushered in decades of debate over how to keep the nation's churches relevant and vital.
>
> Traditional believers, both Protestant and Catholic, have not necessarily thrived in this environment . . . The leaders of [liberal Protestantism] don't seem to be offering anything you can't already get from a purely secular liberalism. Which suggests that perhaps they should pause, amid their frantic renovations, and consider not just what they would change about historic Christianity, but what they would defend and offer uncompromisingly to the world. Absent such a reconsideration, their fate is nearly certain: they will change, and change, and die.[7]

Such critics rarely address the extent to which evangelicals themselves have shifted their own attitudes, reflecting a parallel process of "change, and change, and change." On some social issues such as civil rights, White Evangelicals have shifted their position to reflect perspectives advocated by mainline Protestants decades earlier. On other issues, they have adopted more conservative positions. Throughout the 1980s, the nation's largest Evangelical Protestant denomination, the Southern Baptist Convention, went through a bitter fight between moderates and fundamentalists regarding control of denominational bodies, boards, and institutions.[8] The fundamentalists won and the shift in the denomination has been striking.

The sociologist Mark Chaves has noted a nearly universal trend among the 83 American Protestant bodies he studied toward an internal secularization, a phenomenon he describes as a declining scope of power on the part of religious authorities within a denomination. He notes only one exception among the 83: Southern Baptists. Chaves notes that

> the well-publicized and dramatic recent conflicts within the SBC [Southern Baptist Convention] make clear that this conflict can best be understood as a successful attempt by the religious authority structure to regain control over that denomination's agency structure. The story of the SBC not only illustrates that internal secularization can be reversed, it shows how it can be reversed. A religious authority structure that has lost control over denominational organizational resources can win back that control through political activity.[9]

Over the course of the 1980s, fundamentalists in the Southern Baptist leadership did indeed win back control. A short survey of the Southern Baptists' position on ecumenical cooperation for foreign missions and on the issue of abortion in the United States demonstrates how far the denomination has shifted under fundamentalist control.

Southern Baptists were lukewarm to the ecumenical cooperation that characterized Protestants in the interwar years and following World War II. In the United States, the denomination declined membership in the Federal Council of Churches or its successor the National Council of Churches. Internationally, Southern Baptists declined membership in the World Council of Churches as well. But Southern Baptists did display an openness to international, ecumenical cooperation in some instances. In 1905, Southern Baptists played a key role in the formation of the Baptist World Alliance in London; today, that body has active ties to the World Council of Churches. Southern Baptists also participated in the International Missionary Council, a global Protestant body focused on foreign missions, from the time of its founding in 1921.[10] In 1945, the Baptist Joint Conference on Public Relations, a government advocacy body supported by Southern Baptists, was an enthusiastic participant in efforts to lobby United States delegates to support the Human Rights Commission and the adoption of the Universal Declaration of Human Rights within the United Nations.[11]

The denomination shifted its position to the right over time. In 1961, the International Missionary Council joined the World Council of Churches and participation by Southern Baptists at that point declined sharply. In 2004, Southern Baptists cut ties with the Baptist World Alliance, citing its liberal positions.[12] The attitude of Southern Baptists toward national and international Protestant bodies is reflected in a memorandum on Interdenominational Relationships and presented to the Great Commission Council of the denomination. The memorandum spells out the Southern Baptists' position on ecumenical partnerships and specifically describes both the World Council of Churches and the National Council of Churches:

> Southern Baptists rejected calls for structural unity and declined membership in the National Council of Churches and the World Council of Churches. This has proved to be most wise, for those two councils have fulfilled the worst fears of the Southern Baptists who first declined to join them. A "sham union" has come to characterize these two councils and the larger ecumenical movement. Both are now in captivity to their most radical and liberal elements, and both have rejected biblical Christianity in favor of a modern post-Christian apostasy. The councils have moved from a "lowest common denominator" of theological conviction to the outright repudiation of the Gospel itself.[13]

On the question of abortion, Southern Baptists have also shifted sharply to the right. In 1971, messengers to the annual meeting of the denomination passed a resolution on abortion which read in part, "we call upon Southern Baptists to work for legislation that will allow the possibility of abortion under such conditions as rape, incest, clear evidence of severe fetal deformity, and carefully ascertained evidence of the likelihood of damage to the emotional, mental, and physical health of the mother."[14] In 1974, a year after the Supreme Court issued its legal decision making abortion legal across the nation, messengers reaffirmed the 1971 resolution. Since those two resolutions were approved over 40 years ago, Southern Baptists have since passed 48 other resolutions which reference abortion; of the 50 in total, 22 have abortion or the phrase "the sanctity of human life" in the resolution title and 12 refer sexual and reproductive health issues more broadly in the title.[15] The first five resolutions (from 1971 to 1979) demonstrate nuanced positions while revealing differences in focus; beginning with the 1980 resolution in calling for abortion to be outlawed the resolutions are unequivocal in their position.

Southern Baptists are the largest Protestant denomination in the United States today and they explicitly reject a vision of Christian faith exemplified by bodies such as the World Council of Churches and the National Council of Churches. Their demographic strength in the United States when compared to mainline Protestant denominations means that they have far more social power to influence politics in the United States and the clear consensus they show on social issues reveals their commitment to doing so.

Of course, Southern Baptists are not the only denomination that comprises Evangelicalism, merely the largest. And of course there are nuanced positions on religion and politics among Evangelicals. The sociological shift among Evangelicals and exemplified by Southern Baptists has also influenced Protestant foreign missions more broadly. In 1953, at the height of American religiosity typified by Eisenhower's civil religion and largely communicated through mainline Protestant channels, 18,599 Americans served as career foreign missionaries with just over 50% sponsored by liberal Protestant organizations, 44% sponsored by evangelical bodies and 6% sponsored by bodies affiliated with both liberal and evangelical groups. 1980 saw 35,211 Americans working abroad in foreign missions careers. Of those, 32,101 were sponsored by evangelicals, 3,116 were sponsored by mainline bodies, and only six were sponsored by bodies that aligned with both evangelical and mainline groups; evangelical foreign missionaries outnumber mainline missionaries ten to one, and there were no longer any bodies working across the evangelical/liberal divide.[16]

For Americans both secular and religious who occupied the political mainstream of the 1970s, the rise of evangelicalism in American culture was unexpected. Anthropologist Susan Harding demonstrates just how unexpected it was in her description of the announcement by the fundamentalist[17] Baptist preacher Jerry Falwell in 1979 that he had founded a new political organization called the Moral Majority:

> The reaction of secular Americans, most of whom were themselves religious, to Falwell's announcement, or rather to the sea change in the political scene that his iconic figure and the organization's audacious name telegraphed, was huge . . . Something had just happened we thought was impossible, something that violated the basic tenets of modern history. Both our common sense and our intellectual theories had assured us for several decades that people like Falwell—fundamentalist preachers and their church folk—were disappearing, soon to be extinct, incapable of surviving in a world increasingly ruled by reason and science. Suddenly, it seemed, "they were back."Their coming back not only shocked us, it took something away from us, something more than our sense of which way history was headed. For it turned out that who we were as secular Americans somehow depended on our assumptions about who they were. If "they" weren't dying out as social category, "we" no longer represented the natural, normal, secularizing outcome of modern history. "We" no longer owned the future.[18]

Evangelicals had long avoided engagement in the broader society which was seen as misguided at best and dangerous at worst. This separatist impulse meant that Evangelicals kept a distance from politics. But beginning in the early 1980s, evangelicals began to leverage their numerical, sociological, and economic power to influence government priorities and policies. From the 1980s into the present, the influences of evangelical Protestantism on global health and development began to be more clearly felt not only in regard to foreign missions but also in the foreign policy of the U.S government.

A political analysis of efforts by Evangelical advocates under President George W. Bush to ensure that faith-based organizations could access government funds to carry out social programs including global health and development initiatives documented the complexity and the political messiness of such efforts as these debates moved forward both within the administration and within the U.S. Congress. That analysis is contained in the book *Of Little Faith: The Politics of George W. Bush's Faith-Based Initiatives.*[19] The authors thoroughly document the political wrangling involved in the efforts to enact policy on this topic, analyzing the issues from evangelical perspectives. They raise pointed critiques and they provide a nuanced analysis of their own position. What they never do, however, in over 300 pages is address the Social Gospel, mainline Protestantism, or liberal Protestantism. In short, they employ an entirely different conceptual and critical framework from the one set forth in this book. My point is not to argue for my position over theirs but to demonstrate that Evangelical Christians have developed other intellectual theories, theological positions, and social critiques to make their case and in America today they have amassed greater political capital for implementing policies in the federal government based on their positions.

Cultural shifts in Roman Catholicism

> *To receive in truth the Body and Blood of Christ given up for us, we must recognize Christ in the poorest, his brethren.*
>
> — Catechism of the Catholic Church[20]

Roman Catholicism has been a powerful religious institution in the United States since the colonial era. This book has not focused on Roman Catholicism because the institutional power of Protestantism has played out socially and politically to influence America's global health and development initiatives for over two centuries. Roman Catholicism has not had a similar impact in America's history due to anti-Catholic sentiment. In fact, that sentiment has been part of the social and political influence of Protestantism since the dawn of the American revolution.

The first official act of the Continental Congress—the governmental body that represented the American colonists on governmental matters in relation to the British Parliament—was to protest the passage of the Quebec Act by the Parliament in 1774. That act guaranteed freedom of worship to Roman Catholics under English rule in the Quebec province of the Canadian colonies.[21] Anti-Catholic sentiment was explicit and unabashed in 1928 when Al Smith became the first Roman Catholic nominee for President but such sentiments pervaded other political issues at local, state, and regional levels throughout the 1920s.[22] Anti-Catholic sentiment transcended the long-established liberal/conservative divides of Protestants:

> Despite their own profound theological differences, mainline and evangelical Protestants united in antipathy towards the Church of Rome. Their reasons varied somewhat. The mainline saw the Catholic Church as a totalitarian threat to political and religious liberty, while evangelicals also dismissed Catholicism as superstitious and heretical. Neither camp welcomed Catholic influence in the United States. Both wanted American foreign policy to curb Catholic influence abroad.[23]

In 1950, *The Christian Century*, the weekly magazine that represented the voice of mainline Protestantism, wrote on its editorial pages:

> The United States, through the working of that providence which we call history, is the principal political power engaged in struggle with Russian communism. Naturally, with the Roman church and the American government fighting the same foe, each has tried to make use of the other. In power struggles, such a reaching out after any and every available ally always takes place. Thus the holy war pursued by the papal church and the cold war carried on by the American state have tended to merge . . . It needs to be remembered, however, that the Roman church always has its own purposes, which it never for an instant forgets or surrenders, and that these always involve its own eventual aggrandizement. The Roman church is not only out to defeat its enemies; it is also out to extend its own spiritual authority and ecclesiastical power over all the earth . . . Is America, [European Protestants] are asking, while it says it is fighting a cold war for its own political and social ends, also fighting a holy war for the achievement of Vatican ambitions?[24]

In 1960, after John F. Kennedy defeated Richard Nixon to become the nation's first Roman Catholic President, L. Nelson Bell wrote Nixon. Bell—a former medical missionary to China, father-in-law to American evangelist Billy Graham, and one of the publishers of the evangelical Protestant magazine, *Christianity Today*—was distraught:

> Bell hinted darkly at a more sinister reason for Nixon's loss to John F. Kennedy: "But for the behind-the-scenes organizations (political and religious) you would have won overwhelmingly." Bell's post-script made his reference clear, as he warned of "what is taking place . . . a slow, completely integrated and planned attempt to take over our nation for the Roman Catholic Church." This left Bell despondent: "I feel that the judgment of God hangs over a people to whom He has given so much and who have rejected spiritual values for

> those which are material." The worst fears of Bell and many other Protestants seemed to be coming to pass. America faced spiritual defeat, not by an external atheistic threat, but at the hands of infidels within its own house.[25]

Roman Catholicism gained greater social power in the United States in the last half of the twentieth century. The Catholic church also went through a tumultuous attempt to articulate the church's relationship to the modern world in the Second Vatican Council, or Vatican II, held from 1962–1965. The Council was revolutionary in its support of changes to Roman Catholic worship, advocacy for increased involvement of women, recognition of the contributions of Catholics outside of Western societies, and articulation of a position of engagement with other religious traditions. Gregory Baum was one of the most influential North American Catholic theologians involved in many of the Vatican II meetings. He described the Council glowingly, calling it "'the most powerful spiritual experience I've had in all my life' . . . Bishops and theologians 'were open to new ideas, and people were anxious to make Christianity [and] the Gospel understandable to people today. Great things happened.' "[26] Despite his appreciation for spirit of Vatican II, Baum also bemoaned the lost opportunities represented by the failure of the church to fully act on the ideas and spirit that came out of the meetings, claiming that any efforts to understand the church and the conflicts it faces today "must take into consideration the decision of Rome to renege on the promises of Vatican II and the as yet unresolved theological problems produced by the teaching of Vatican II."[27]

Religious traditions other than Christianity

Christianity has never been the sole religion in America—merely the one that is most socially pervasive. The first Jewish congregation in the United States, Shearith Israel, was established in New Amsterdam in 1654, predating the renaming of the city by 20 years, when the British seized control in 1674.[28] (For data on the number of Jews in America, see Table 7.5) The first Muslims in America were slaves from West Africa. Records of Muslim slaves date back to the eighteenth century. After the abolition of slavery, Muslim immigrants began arriving in small numbers in the 1870s, but it would take another 40 years for Muslim communities to grow in size in order to establish the first known mosque in Biddeford, Maine in 1915.[29] (For data on number of Muslims in America, see Table 7.5.). Though they do not match Christian organizations when comparing overall budgets, two of the 20 largest faith-based organizations in the United States according to 2015 revenues were American Jewish World Service (AJWS) and Islamic Relief U.S. AJWS was the 20th largest with total revenues of $58,158,816 and Islamic Relief was 12th largest with a budget of $110,899,089. Neither receives any funds from the United States government whereas many of the other top twenty organizations (all Christian) do.

Among those who received no U.S. government funds, Islamic Relief was third and AJWS was sixth.[30]

No religious involvement at all: America's fast growing religious demographic

If Judaism and Islam were parts of the nation's religious fabric—albeit in small numbers—for centuries, many nonetheless assume that the lack of religious involvement was uncommon in the United States until the secular turn in the 1960s. This is actually not the case; in fact, religious participation in America has ebbed and flowed over the years. At the dawn of the American Revolution in 1776, only 17% of the population maintained church membership. By 1850 in the years after the Second Great Awakening, that percentage was 34%. The third chapter of this book opens with a description of the work of William Gorgas, an early public health pioneer who worked to eradicate tropical disease. Gorgas was not a particularly religious man and there are no references in the biographical materials on Gorgas that point to religion playing any important role in his life. The religious life of Gorgas' father, however, illuminates the tensions between faith and doubt and the social expectations to practice religion in the nineteenth century nonetheless:

> I am but an indifferent church-goer, and prefer staying at home to read and write. Were I lucky enough to hear a preacher occasionally whose sermon gave me something to think about, I should doubtless attend worship oftener. The religious principal is however not very strong in me. . . . It is Sunday and I ought to have gone to church, the bells for which are now ringing reproachfully, but I did not feel like it, a poor excuse I fear. In consequence of my defection, Minnie is also at home. If we were members we should feel ourselves compelled to attend more regularly, and after all it is a good thing to have a day set apart for something besides making money, or doing work, something a little more intellectual, if not religious. I do not however like to go day after day and make professions which do not come wholly from the heart, and which are but too frequently accompanied by a yawn. How many hundreds of times have I gone over the service of the Episcopal Church, and yet I cannot repeat twenty consecutive words in it, beyond the Lord's prayer! Yet it is better to attend church regularly even if we do not join in the services. I have often there heard words which made me think, and not infrequently made me for the time being a better man. If we but listen to an earnest, honest man in the pulpit we are not wasting our time. This at least we can do without that feeling of self-doubting, which strikes me when I join in a service which is but too often to me only words, words, words, most unprofitably spoken. . . .

> The day is beautiful, and the air pleasant. It is Sunday & I attended church this morning. I omitted to state that Mamma and I were baptized and confirmed on the same day (Tuesday May 6, 1862). [Confederate] President Jefferson Davis and one other person were the only others confirmed, the confirmation being held by the bishop for him. . . . My mind has since turned oftener toward religious thoughts, and I trust I shall benefit by thus linking myself to the visible church.[31]

Gorgas maintained his ties to the Episcopal Church, eventually serving as a Vice-Chancellor at Sewanee, an Episcopal college in Tennessee, before becoming President of the University of Alabama. His diary is striking not for any particular revelation regarding religion and global health but because it demonstrates both a personal struggle with religious belief and a social obligation to participate in religious practice. This dynamic has always been part of religion in any society, including the United States.[32]

The resiliency of this dynamic has led to revision of a perspective common among sociologists in the late 1960s. The perspective that Americans and Europeans were abandoning religious institutions became known as the secularization thesis. Peter Berger is an American sociologist who famously articulated the secularization thesis in his 1967 book *The Sacred Canopy: Elements of a Sociological Theory of Religion*. Berger is also the most famous of the early champions of secularization thesis to recant his claim. He argues that modernity is characterized not by the absence of God but by a competition of many gods vying for our allegiance. Modernity, says Berger, is not secularizing but pluralizing.[33]

Proponents of secularization argue that scientific knowledge presents insights and data that are fundamentally irreconcilable with religious belief; thus, the assumption goes, education levels will have an inverse relationship to religiosity with scientists emerging as the clear-eyed skeptics of religion. In fact, this has not been the case. In 1916, the psychologist James Leuba conducted a study to measure religious belief among eminent scientists and found that 41.8% expressed a belief in a God "to whom one may pray in the expectation of receiving an answer."[34] In 1997, two scholars repeated his study, employing the same wording in the survey and drawing study participants from the same source. 39.3% of study respondents expressed a belief in God using the exact same definition.[35] Over that 100 year span, religious belief in God had remained steady among scientists, according to the study. In fact, there is some indication that religiosity is higher among scientists than humanities scholars. Commenting on the 1997 study in *The New York Times*, sociologist Rodney Stark noted that

> teachers of the so-called hard sciences, like math and chemistry, are more likely to be devout than are professors of such softer sciences as anthropology and psychology or of the humanities. . . . The reason for the discrepancy may be

> that, in an odd sort of way, traditional religious dogma suits the mathematically inclined mind, suggested George Marsden, a professor of religious history. . . . "It could be that scientists are used to looking for definite answers, whereas humanists go into their field because they like to deal with ambiguities."[36]

The preoccupation with the existential question of religious belief minimizes the question of social context in relation to religious belief and doubt. While Josiah Gorgas could only write about his doubts in his private journal, a growing percentage of Americans no longer feel a need to maintain an outward veneer of religious piety while finding little useful in organized religion. As of 2008, 34 million Americans, or 15% of the adult population, identified no religious affiliation when surveyed by the American Religious Identity Survey (see Table 7.5). And in 2014, the U.S. Religious Landscape Study by the Pew Research Center on Religion and Public Life found that Americans unaffiliated with any religion tradition had grown from 16.1% of the population in 2007 to 22.8% while those who identified as Christian fell from 78.4% to 70.6% (with reductions in percentage occurring among Mainline and Evangelical Protestants as well as Roman Catholics).[37]

This lowered social pressure to acknowledge religiosity is not equivalent to secularization because it does not reflect a loss of belief in God per se, though it does demonstrate a loss of religion's capacity to serve as a driver of social cohesion. Even among the religiously unaffiliated, however, personal belief in God is still high, albeit lower than in the population overall. Over half of the "No Religion" respondents in the 2008 American Religious Identity Survey affirmed a belief in either a higher power or a personal God, while 7% stated that they did not believe that God existed (see Table 7.5). In the 2014 Religious Landscape Report, the percentage of American identifying as atheist grew from 1.6 to 3.1 from 2007 to 2014 while those identifying as agnostic grew from 2.4 to 4.0% in the same period.[38]

The implications of America's shifting religious landscape on global health and development

America's religious landscape is vastly different from that of a century ago when the Social Gospel represented the priorities of American Protestants. While religious observance in the United States remains far higher in comparison to Canada and Europe, those with no religious affiliation represent the largest and fastest growing demographic in relation to religion. The foreign missions activities of Evangelical Protestants and Roman Catholics in the United States have always influenced American notions of global health and development but their greater numbers now represent a social force that has upended the singular role that mainline Protestants played a century ago. Further, the increased social and political power of Evangelical Protestants and Roman Catholics have influenced the foreign policy priorities

Table 7.5 Number of Jewish and Muslim Americans and Americans indicating no religious affiliation.

	1990 (#s in thousands)				2001 (#s in thousands)				2008 (#s in thousands)			
	Number	Increase/ (Decrease)	% Change	% US adult pop (175,440)	Number	Increase/ (Decrease)	% Change	% US adult pop (207,983)	Number	Increase/ (Decrease)	% Change	% US adult pop (228,182)
Judaism	3,137	N/A	N/A	1.8%	2,831	(306)	–9.6%	1.4%	2,680	(151)	–5.8%	1.2%
Muslim	527	N/A	N/A	.3%	1,104	577	109.5%	.5%	1,349	245	22.2%	.6%
Christianity	151,225	N/A	N/A	86.2%	159,514	8,289	5.5%	76.7%	173,402	13,888	8.7%	76.0%
No Religion	14,331	N/A	N/A	8.2%	29,481	15,150	105.7%	14.2%	34,169	4,688	15.9%	15.0%

Characteristics of "Nones"

Researchers at The American Religious Identification Survey define Nones as a label for a diverse group of people who do not identify with any of the myriad of religious options in the American religious marketplace—the irreligious, the unreligious, the anti-religious, and the anti-clerical. Some believe in God; some do not. Some may participate occasionally in religious rituals; others never will. The researchers also found the following:

- "Nones" are not a stable demographic group. 41% of those who identify as "none" at the age of 12 are part of a religious tradition in adulthood.
- Nonetheless, "Nones" are growing more rapidly as a percentage of all Americans. The number of Americans who identified as part of some religious tradition in 1990 but had become a "None" by 2008 was 11% of the nation's population. The number of Americans who identified as "None" in 1990 but had become part of some religious tradition by 2008 was 4% of the population.
- "Nones" do not all reject a belief in God. The following table shows responses to the question, "Regarding the existence of God, do you think. . . ."

Response	*Category*	*Percentage Nones (N=1,106)*	*Percentage US Adults (N=1,015)*
There is no such thing	Atheist	7	2
There is no way to know	Hard Agnostic	19	4
I'm not sure	Soft Agnostic	16	6
There is a higher power but no personal God	Deist	24	12
There is definitely a personal God	Theist	27	70
Don't know/Refused	N/A	7	6

Source: Statistical Abstract of the United States, 2012.

of the American government in relation to international health and development in different ways from the influence that Mainline Protestants exerted.

Modern Roman Catholic social teaching can provide a foundation for partnership with global health and development programs; it can also reveal tensions. The modern-day articulation of Catholic social teaching traces back to the late nineteenth century and is drawn from doctrinal statements, papal encyclicals, and documents from church councils.[39] Over the last 125 years, the Church has developed a cohesive body of social teaching that articulates the church's position on social issues. The U.S. Conference of Catholic Bishops (USCCB) authorized a committee to develop materials for teaching American Catholics about the church's social thought, and in 1998, it published a summary report on that committee's efforts. In the document, the USCCB lays out seven themes:

- *The Life and Dignity of the Human Person*. This belief is the foundation of all subsequent social teaching because "each person is precious, people are more important than things, and the measure of every institution is whether it threatens or enhances the life and dignity of the human person." Drawing upon this point of view, the Bishops challenge abortion, assisted suicide, human cloning and genetic engineering.
- *Call to Family, Community, and Participation*. This theme argues that human beings are created by God to be social creatures and the ways we organize ourselves socially through economics, politics, and law has a direct effect on human dignity. As the central social institutions, the family must be supported and strengthened. The Bishops challenge individualism and claim that people have both a right and a responsibility to participate in society and to seek the common good by attending especially to the poor and vulnerable.
- *Rights and Responsibilities*. Human beings must find the proper balance between the rights they legitimately enjoy and the responsibilities placed before them to use those rights to support their families, communities, and the larger society.
- *Option for the Poor and Vulnerable*. While tremendous wealth is a reality for some, it is often secured through systems that entrench pervasive poverty as a social reality for most. Societies must work to ensure that vulnerable members are faring well and progressing. "Our tradition recalls the story of the Last Judgment and instructs us to put the needs of the poor and vulnerable first."
- *The Dignity of Work and The Rights of Workers*. The bishops argue that economies should be structured to serve people and not people made to serve economies. Work should not only be tied to earning a living but to participation in God's creation. For this to happen, workers' rights must be protected.
- *Solidarity*. Modern society tempts us to turn inward. However, "we are our brothers' and sisters' keepers, wherever they live." Solidarity reminds us that loving our neighbor has taken on global significance in our world today.

- *Care for God's Creation*. Human beings respect the Creator through faithful stewardship of the creation. Such stewardship obligates us to consider politics, policies, and economics in addition to our daily practices and habits.[40]

The Catholic theological ethicist Lisa Sowle Cahill argues that these teachings enable a Roman Catholic approach to global health and development:

> At the international level, Catholic organizations . . . are active in trying to provide health-related services and to change worldwide spending patterns and national and international policies. A key example is Catholic involvement in international activism around the AIDS crisis, both to provide services to AIDS victims and to advocate making patented drugs available at lower prices for lower-income persons and nations. Although the Catholic Church is probably better known for its opposition to the use of condoms to prevent HIV transmission, it is equally true that the church is the single greatest provider of services to AIDS victims in the world. Vatican spokesmen have also publicly criticized international trade rules that prevent access to life-saving drugs for AIDS and other diseases . . . In 2004, a Vatican representative excoriated international pharmaceutical companies whose patents, protected by the World Trade Organization, keep the price of necessary drugs out of reach of the poor.
>
> A Catholic ethic for global health care must respect the dignity and empower the agency of all those affected by poverty and disease. It must involve local, regional, national, international, transnational, and global actors to act in solidarity with those who suffer. And it must mobilize Catholics at every level to act for the global common good by affirming health care as a Christian duty and a human right and by adopting the option for the poor as the first step toward global health justice.[41]

Catholic social teaching is also informed by the tradition of liberation theology, a tradition rooted in reflection on the Scriptures and church teachings by local communities across Central and South America. Gustavo Gutierrez is one of the best known voices in liberation theology and is often credited with helping to articulate key elements of the tradition, especially the notion of God's preferential option for the poor, which Gutierrez laid out in his 1973 book, *A Theology of Liberation*. In 2011, Gutierrez sat with Paul Farmer, Chair of Global Health and Social Medicine at the Harvard Medical School and the founder of the health and development organization Partners in Health. That discussion formed the basis for a book on liberation theology and global health entitled *In the Company of the Poor: Conversations with Dr. Paul Farmer and Fr. Gustavo Gutierrez*.

In the book, the two men explore the implications of the idea of God's preferential option for the poor and describe the challenge and rewards of building an honest relationship with those who are poor based not on pity or the demands of a funder, or the effort to meet program objectives. They describe the value of relationship with people who are poor because they are, first and foremost, people and knowing them as people in their own social location can reveal to those of us from wealthier societies our participation in the sinful social structures that create, sustain, and embed poverty as a way of life for too many people around the global. Creating, building, and caring for this relationship is the process that Gutierrez describes as accompaniment.

Reflecting on the discussions between Farmer and Gutierrez and the implications for this relationship of accompaniment for global health and development, Steve Reifenberg, a professor of development studies at Notre Dame, wrote:

> Envisioning international development aid as "accompaniment"—that we're in this together, and not just for a little while, but for the long run—would call us to identify and support institutions that truly represent the poor; partner with public institutions rather than "go it alone"; make job creation a benchmark of success; invest directly in the poor themselves; and establish learning loops that put in practice what we learn through this accompaniment process. "True accompaniment does not privilege technical expertise above solidarity, compassion, and a willingness to tackle what may seem insuperable challenges," writes Farmer. "It requires cooperation, openness, and humility; this concept may, I hope, infuse new vitality into development work."[42]

Catholic social teaching provides a basis for faith-inspired global health and development work today. But Catholic theology also complicates some aspects of that work, particularly in relation to sexual and reproductive health. This is to say to the two ways of understanding sexual practices drawn from the field of global health and from the field of Catholic moral theology are in certain aspects in some level of fundamental tension with each other. That tension will not dissipate by appeals to data or outcomes on the part of the health researcher or practitioner or by a recitation of moral principles embedded within Catholic social teaching. They represent, rather, two different ways of thinking about sexual practices and health. As profound as Catholic social principles are and as radically faithful as liberation theology is as a foundation for sustained health and development work, Roman Catholic moral theological teaching against the use of a condom as a barrier device to prevent HIV infection stands at odds with sound HIV prevention research and practice.

The position any one of us takes on the poles of this tension of course depends, of course, on what we prioritize. The fact is that countless numbers of practicing Roman Catholics also support comprehensive HIV prevention efforts or work in global health programs where condoms are distributed speaks to the negotiations they make as individuals across this divide but it does not erase the fact of the divide on the social level. Catholicism, like Protestantism—in fact, like all religions—displays elements of strong alignment with health and development and elements of tension.

Other religious voices have also impacted the ways in which religion influences international health and development. Researchers in the field of global health and development who study religion have debated how to understand the influence of religion in their field and to define the kinds of organizations in health and development practice that are motivated by religious belief. These debates have revealed the ways in which the long-standing collaboration with Christian organizations in these fields has limited understanding of other organizational structures and the influences of other religious traditions.[43]

The challenges in efforts to better understand the relationship between religious traditions other than Christianity and global health and development are not limited to questions of organizational structures, however. Global politics, especially since September 11, impact the ways in which Islam is examined in this field and have contributed to tensions between global health and development programs and programs designed to address potential threats to health and well-being. One key challenge in this context is to correctly measure religion's influence. On the one hand, some have critiqued analyses of this religious extremism that frame it as a "clash of civilizations" between the Christian west and the Muslim middle east.[44] In contrast, others have rejected any equivalency between the religious ideology of violent extremism in Islam and the practice of the religion among the vast majority of its adherents.[45] Nonetheless, most Islamic charities have faced close scrutiny of their finances, with governments (most often from the U.S. and Europe) looking for any money trails by which charities are financing violent extremism in the guise of humanitarian aid.[46]

Such scrutiny has created enormous challenges for any form of humanitarian work to be carried out in some countries with Muslim majorities—even that sponsored by Christian or secular groups—because of suspicion of aid efforts as disguised surveillance by Western governments.[47] Such challenges are not limited to carrying out global health and development in parts of the world in need of such programs. In Chapter 6, we examined the ways in which the threat of nuclear war impacted public health efforts in the United States using an analysis by the anthropologist Joseph Masco. In fact, Masco argues that a similar cultural framework has been used to fight the "war on terror":

> The effects of [conceptualizing health not as absence of disease but as avoiding an ever-present danger of death] in the logics of health and national security are still with us today. The reactions to the suicide attacks[48] on Washington, DC and New York in 2001 reinvigorated the emotional management strategy and returned Americans to the logics of survival and sacrifice that structured the Cold War period. The threat of terrorism was, in fact, magnified by the George W. Bush administration into grounds for a fundamental rethinking of

> U.S. global ambitions as well as U.S. domestic policy, just as the first Soviet nuclear test in 1949 was mobilized by the Truman and Eisenhower administrations to construct the Cold War state. The state's appeal to citizens after 2001 was also modeled on the early civil defense campaigns as it argued for a normalization rather than an elimination of a totalized threat.[49]

Finally, the debates over secularization often create an either/or dynamic between champions of religion's contributions to global health and development and critics of religion who see it complicating health and development efforts. On the one hand, advocates for the contributions of religion articulate strong positions on religion's positive impact, assuming that the rabid secularity of present-day global health and development practitioners has blinded them to the influences of religion. Such efforts run the risk of minimizing or overlooking the ways in which religion complicates health and development practices. On the other hand, critics of religion describe religion's complicating influences without much attention to its contributions.

An example of the former is found in the groundbreaking 2007 report by researchers in the African Religious Health Assets Programme working with the World Health Organization to map religious health assets in Sub-Saharan Africa. The report sets the tone in its very first lines:

> Though often hidden from Western view, religion is so overwhelmingly significant in the African search for well-being, so deeply woven in the rhythms of everyday life, and so deeply entwined in African values, attitudes, perspectives and decision-making frameworks that the inability to understand religion leads to an inability to understand people's lives.

The report begins with an assumption that global health programs fail to consider religion even though the project was funded by the World Health Organization. Having started with this assumption, the report goes on to articulate an enthusiastic case for the distinctive value of "religious health assets" while never seriously considering the ways in which religion may contribute to poorer health outcomes.[50] An example of the latter is found in a report examining the influence of religion on global HIV programs for communities facing stigma such as men who have sex with men, sex workers, and people who use drugs. The Executive Summary of that report argues for a global response to HIV "that is grounded in science—and not religious ideology—and that advances the human rights of lesbian, gay, bisexual, and transgender, or LGBT, populations as well as other specific subpopulations."[51] In arguing that religion is a driver of stigma for some marginalized populations most affected by HIV—a claim that is unquestionably true—the report fails to consider that religion may actually motivate both compassion and sound public health practice for these communities as well.

The religious landscape in America has indeed shifted and those shifts impact health and development programs and priorities in ways far different from the influences of foreign missions' initiatives enlivened by the Social Gospel. The transfer of the empire of the world is being carried out through religious traditions other than American Protestantism. In the retreat of this liberal Protestantism, a certain brand of evangelicalism has filled the vacuum to author and interpret America's civil religion. It emerged out of its exile after the fundamentalist-modernist controversies of the 1920s and 30s much more conservative and emboldened to be overtly political. Some of the most overtly political expressions of American evangelicalism are at odds with other religious movements in America. This tension shows up in Roman Catholic social teaching, a chastened mainline Protestantism that now supports far more prophetic positions, Black church traditions, Judaism, Islam, some branches of evangelicalism itself, the spiritual practices of the religious "nones," and a growing number of agnostics and atheists. Each of these groups will have something to say about the rhetoric of a civil religion in America and they will add their own perspectives regarding the political priorities and practices such rhetoric will be used to justify.

The question—unknown and unknowable at this point in time because it is only now unfolding—is whether evangelical Protestantism will articulate the narrative of its own tensions or whether it will re-articulate a triumphalist, nationalistic American Christianity. That is the ethical, moral, and political battle currently being waged within the movement. Short-term wins are not an indication of victory at the level of the culture. After all, liberal Protestantism after World War I was bold enough to preach with confidence that its vision of global peace was just around the corner when less than a decade later it was experiencing a crisis of confidence and a second, devastating world war began to unfold. Will evangelicalism retreat from its current political niche as it reckons with the implications of political actions that it finds unconscionable are carried out in its name? Or will it double down on its power? As it faces moral crises—and they will come—how will it respond?

Notes

1 Albert Mohler, "Where Have all the Liberals Gone? – The Riverside Church Seeks New Pastor," albertmohler.com, May 9, 2007, www.albertmohler.com/2007/05/09/where-have-all-the-liberals-gone-the-riverside-church-seeks-new-pastor/, accessed February 28, 2018.

2 "Protest to Eisenhower: Group Asks Him to Reconsider Speech to Church Council," *The New York Times*, August 7, 1954, p. 14.

3 NCC Press Release, September 10, 1956. Cited in William Inboden, *Religion and American Foreign Policy 1945–1960: The Soul of Containment* (New York: Cambridge University Press, 2008), 71.

4 Ibid., p. 74.

5 Inboden explores this at length. See pp. 81–99.

6 Ibid., p. 274.

7 Ross Douthat, "Can Liberal Christianity Be Saved?" *The New York Times*, p. SR11, July 15, 2012.

8 For a thorough and accessible history of these events, see Nancy Ammerman, *Baptist Battles: Social Change and Religious Conflict in the Southern Baptist Convention* (New Brunswick, NJ: Rutgers University Press, 1990).

9 Mark Chaves, "Interorganizational Power and Internal Secularization in Protestant Denominations," in *The American Journal of Sociology* 99, no. 1 (1993), 38–39.

10 H. Cornell Goerner, "World Missions After the War," in *Review and Expositor* 40, no 3 (1943): 319–331.

11 John Nurser, "The 'Ecumenical Movement' Churches, 'Global Order,' and Human Rights: 1938–1948," in *Human Rights Quarterly* 25, no. 4 (2003): 2003.

12 Alan Cooperman, "Southern Baptists Vote to Leave World Alliance," in *The Washington Post*, June 16, 2004, A12.

13 Albert Mohler, *The Southern Baptist Convention and the Issue of Interdenominational Partnerships* (memorandum, Louisville, KY, 2009), Online: https://albertmohler.com/2009/07/16/the-southern-baptist-convention-and-the-issue-of-interdenominational-relationships/, accessed March 7, 2018.

14 Southern Baptist Convention, *Resolution on Abortion* (resolution, St. Louis, MO, 1971), www.sbc.net/resolutions/13/resolution-on-abortion, accessed March 7, 2018.

15 For a searchable database of all resolutions passed by the Southern Baptist Convention, go to www.sbc.net/resolutions/search/

16 Robert T. Coote, "The Uneven Growth of Conservative Evangelical Missions," in *International Bulletin of Missionary Research* 6, no. 3 (1982): 120.

17 In fact, evangelicalism and fundamentalist Christianity are not the same thing theologically. In many parts of the world, they are not the same sociologically; in the United States, however, strong ties have been built between evangelicals and fundamentalist Christians over the last four decades.

18 Susan F. Harding, "American Protestant Moralism and the Secular Imagination: From Temperance to the Moral Majority," in *Social Research* 76, no. 4 (2009): 1277–1278.

19 Amy E. Black, Douglas L. Koopman, and David K. Ryden, *Of Little Faith: The Politics of George W. Bush's Faith-Based Initiatives* (Washington, DC: Georgetown University Press, 2004).

20 Catholic Church. "The Paschal Banquet," in *The Catechism of the Catholic Church*, 2nd ed. (Vatican: Libreria Editrice Vaticana, 2012), www.vatican.va/archive/ENG0015/_P42.HTM, accessed March 5, 2018.

21 Walter A. McDougall, *Promised Land, Crusader State: The American Encounter with the World Since 1776* (New York: Houghton Mifflin, 1997), 18.

22 Lynn Dumenil, "The Tribal Twenties: 'Assimilated' Catholics' Response to Anti-Catholicsm in the 1920s," in *Journal of American Ethnic History* 11, no. 1 (1991): 21–49.

23 William Inboden, *Religion and American Foreign Policy 1945–1960: The Soul of Containment* (New York: Cambridge University Press, 2008), 58–59.

24 "Is the Cold War a Holy War?" in *Unsigned editorial. Christian Century* 67, no. 2 (1950): 41.

25 Inboden, p. 312.

26 Baum was quoted in his obituary, published by National Catholic Reporter. See Heidi Sclumpf, "Gregory Baum, influential theologian of Vatican II era, dies at 94," in *National Catholic Reporter*, October 20, 2017, www.ncronline.org/news/people/gregory-baum-influential-theologian-vatican-ii-era-dies-94, accessed March 5, 2018.

27 Gregory Baum, "The Forgotten Promises of Vatican II," in *Historical Studies* 77 (2011): 22.

28 Jacob R. Marcus, *Early American Jewry: The Jews of New York, New England, and Canada, 1649–1794: Volume I* (Philadelphia: Jewish Publication Society, 1951), 20–23.

29 "Islam in America," The Harvard Pluralism Project, Online: http://pluralism.org/religions/islam/islam-in-america/, accessed March 5, 2018.

30 Jean Duff, *Sources of Revenue and International Expenditures of US Faith-Based NGOs, Based on IRS 990 Forms for Fiscal Years 2011–2015* (Washington, DC: Center for Faith and the Common Good, 2017), 6.

31 Josiah Gorgas, *Journals of Josiah Gorgas, 1857–1878*, Sarah Woolfolk Wiggins, ed. (Tuscaloosa: University of Alabama Press, 2014), 11, 21, 49–50.

32 The sociologist Rodney Stark offers a concise but well-supported argument that European society was not significantly more "Christian" at any point in its history than it is today. He has two points in his argument. The first is that religious membership was never particularly high in Europe, even at the height of the church's political power. The second is that people in Europe

today profess high levels of religious belief even in the absence of widespread corporate religious practice. See Rodney Stark, "Secularization, R.I.P.," in *Sociology of Religion* 60, no. 3 (1999): 249–273.

33 Peter L. Berger, "Secularization Falsified," in *First Things* 180 (2008): 23–27.

34 James Leuba, *The Belief in God and Immortality: A Psychological, Anthropological, and Statistical Study* (Chicago: Open Court Publishers, 1921).

35 Edward J. Larson and Larry Witham, "Scientists are Still Keeping the Faith," in *Nature* 386, no. 6624 (1997): 435–436.

36 Natalie Angier, "Survey of Scientists Finds a Stability of Faith in God," in *The New York Times*, April 3, 1997, p. A 10.

37 Pew Research Center, *America's Changing Religious Landscape* (Washington, DC: Pew Research Center, 2015), Online: http://assets.pewresearch.org/wp-content/uploads/sites/11/2015/05/RLS-08-26-full-report.pdf, accessed March 5, 2018.

38 Ibid.

39 John Coleman, *One Hundred Years of Catholic Social Thought: Celebration and Challenge* (Maryknoll, NY: Orbis, 1991).

40 U.S. Conference of Catholic Bishops, *Sharing Catholic Social Teaching: Challenges and Directions – Reflections of the U.S. Bishops* (Washington, DC: USCCB Publishing, 1998), 4.

41 Lisa Sowle Cahill, "Global Health and Catholic Social Commitment," in *Health Progress* 88, no. 3 (2007): 56–57.

42 Steve Reifenberg, "Afterword," in *In the Company of the Poor: Conversations with Dr. Paul Farmer and Fr. Gustavo Gutierrez*, Michael Griffin and Jennie Weiss Block, eds. (Maryknoll, NY: Orbis, 2013), 195.

43 See Jill Olivier, "'An FB-oh?': Mapping the Etymology of the Religious Entity Engaged in Health," in *When Religion and Health Align: Mobilizing Religious Health Assets for Transformation*, James Cochrane, Barbara Schmid, and Teresa Cutts, eds. (Pietermaritzburg, SA: Cluster Publications, 2011). For a case study on these issues in the context of Hinduism in India, Nalin Mehta and Upahar Pramanik, "HIV and the gurus: religiosity, plurality and the challenge of a 'Hindu" response," in *South Asian History and Culture* 1, no. 2 (2010): 250–267.

44 See, for example, Ervand Abrahamian, "The US media, Huntington and September 11," in *Third World Quarterly* 24, no. 3 (2003): 529–544. There are many sustained critiques such as the one Abrahamian articulates. Many of them critique the thesis put forth by the historian Samuel Huntington that recent violence carried out in the name of Islam reflects as "clash of civilizations."

45 See, for example, Bruno Etienne, "Islam and Violence," in *History and Anthropology* 18, no. 3 (2007): 237–248. Again, there are many sustained analyses comparable to Etienne's.

46 Jonathan Benthall, "Humanitarianism and Islam after 11 September," in *Humanitarian Action and the 'Global War on Terror': A Review of Trends and Issues*, Joanna Macrae and Adele Harmer, eds., pp. 37–48 (London: Humanitarian Policy Group, 2003), 45.

47 Stephen Hopgood and Leslie Vinjamuri, "Faith in Markets," in *Sacred Aid: Faith and Humanitarianism*, Michael Barnett and Janice Gross Stein, eds, pp. 37–64, (London: Oxford University Press, 2012), 44.

48 An important point: at no point in his analysis does Masco refer to religion. This is, to my mind, a weakness in his conceptualization of both "the war on terror" and the nuclear threat of the Cold War.

49 Joseph Masco, "Atomic Health, or How the Bomb Altered American Notions of Death," in *Against Health: How Health Became the New Morality*, Jonathan M. Metzl, and Anna Kirkland, eds., pp. 133–154 (New York: NYU Press, 2010), 149.

50 African Religious Health Assets Programme (ARHAP), *Appreciating Assets: The Contribution of Religion to Universal Access in Africa* (Cape Town: ARHAP, 2007), 1. I am a part of the body that carried out this work, now known as IRHAP – the International Religious Health Assets Programme – and have participated in a variety of research and practice initiatives as part of this organization. The criticism I made regarding the report's overly optimistic assessment of religious health assets would not be new to the members of IRHAP with whom I work.

51 Scott H. Evertz, *How Ideology Trumped Science: How PEPFAR Failed to Meet Its Potential* (Washington: Center for American Progress and the Council for Global Equality, 2010), 3.

References

Abrahamian, Ervand. "The US Media, Huntington and September 11." *ThirdWorld Quarterly* 24, no. 3 (2003): 529–544.

African Religious Health Assets Programme (ARHAP). *Appreciating Assets: The Contribution of Religion to Universal Access in Africa*. Cape Town: ARHAP, 2007.

Ammerman, Nancy. *Baptist Battles: Social Change and Religious Conflict in the Southern Baptist Convention*. New Brunswick, NJ: Rutgers University Press, 1990.

Angier, Natalie. "Survey of Scientists Finds a Stability of Faith in God." *The New York Times*, April 3, 1997, p. A 10.

Baum, Gregory. "The Forgotten Promises of Vatican II." *Historical Studies* 77 (2011): 7–22.

Benthall, Jonathan. "Humanitarianism and Islam After 11 September." In *Humanitarian Action and the 'Global War on Terror': A Review of Trends and Issues*, eds. Joanna Macrae and Adele Harmer. London: Humanitarian Policy Group, 2003, 37–48.

Berger, Peter L. "Secularization Falsified." *First Things* 180 (2008): 23–27.

Black, Amy E., Douglas L. Koopman, and David K. Ryden. *Of Little Faith: The Politics of George W. Bush's Faith-Based Initiatives*. Washington, DC: Georgetown University Press, 2004.

Blevins, John Mimi Kiser, Emily Lemon, and Ahoua Kone. "The Percentage of HIV Treatment and Prevention Services in Kenya Provided by Faith Based Health Providers." *Development in Practice* 27, no. 5 (2017): 646–657.

Blevins, John. "When Sodomy Leads to Martyrdom: Sex, Religion, and Politics in Historical and Contemporary Contexts in Uganda and East Africa," *Theology and Sexuality* 17, no. 1 (2011): 51–74.

Blevins, John and Peter Irungu. "Different Ways of Doing Violence: Sexuality, Religion, and Public Health in Same Gender-Loving Men in Kenya." *The Journal of the American Academy of Religion* 83, no. 4 (2015): 930–946.

Cahill, Lisa Sowle. "Global Health and Catholic Social Commitment." *Health Progress* 88, no. 3 (2007): 56–57.

Catholic Church. "The Paschal Banquet." In *The Catechism of the Catholic Church*, 2nd ed. Vatican: Libreria Editrice Vaticana, 2012, www.vatican.va/archive/ENG0015/_P42.HTM, Accessed March 5, 2018.

Chaves, Mark. "Interorganizational Power and Internal Secularization in Protestant Denominations." *The American Journal of Sociology* 99, no. 1 (1993), 38–39.

Coleman, John. *One Hundred Years of Catholic Social Thought: Celebration and Challenge*. Maryknoll, NY: Orbis, 1991.

Cooperman, Alan. "Southern Baptists Vote to Leave World Alliance." *The Washington Post*, June 16, 2004, p. A12.

Coote, Robert T. "The Uneven Growth of Conservative Evangelical Missions." *International Bulletin of Missionary Research* 6, no. 3 (1982): 118–123.

Douthat, Ross. "Can Liberal Christianity Be Saved?" *The New York Times*, July 15, 2012, p. SR11.

Duff, Jean. *Sources of Revenue and International Expenditures of US Faith-Based NGOs, Based on IRS 990 Forms for Fiscal Years 2011–2015*. Washington, DC: Center for Faith and the Common Good, 2017.

Dumenil, Lynn. "The Tribal Twenties: 'Assimilated' Catholics' Response to Anti- Catholicsm in the 1920s." *Journal of American Ethnic History* 11, no. 1 (1991): 21–49.

Etienne, Bruno. "Islam and Violence." *History and Anthropology* 18, no. 3 (2007): 237–248.

Evertz, Scott H. *How Ideology Trumped Science: How PEPFAR Failed to Meet Its Potential*. Washington: Center for American Progress and the Council for Global Equality, 2010.

Farmer, Paul and Gustavo Gutierrez. *In the Company of the Poor: Conversations with Dr. Paul Farmer and Fr. Gustavo Gutierrez*, eds. Michael Griffin and Jennie Weiss Block. Maryknoll, NY: Orbis, 2013.

Goerner, H. Cornell. "World Missions After the War." *Review and Expositor* 40, no 3 (1943): 319–331.

Gorgas, Josiah. *Journals of Josiah Gorgas, 1857–1878*, ed. Sarah Woolfolk Wiggins. Tuscaloosa: University of Alabama Press, 2014, pp. 11, 21, 49–50.

Harding, Susan F. "American Protestant Moralism and the Secular Imagination: From Temperance to the Moral Majority." Social Research 76, no. 4 (2009): 1277–1306.

Hopgood, Stephen and Leslie Vinjamuri. "Faith in Markets." In *Sacred Aid: Faith and Humanitarianism*, eds. Michael Barnett and Janice Gross Stein, 37–64. London: Oxford University Press, 2012.

Inboden, William. *Religion and American Foreign Policy, 1945–1960: The Soul of Containment*. New York: Cambridge University Press, 2008.

"Is the Cold War a Holy War?" Unsigned editorial. *Christian Century* 67, no. 2 (1950): 39–41.

"Islam in America." The Harvard Pluralism Project. http://pluralism.org/religions/islam/islam-in-america/, Accessed March 5, 2018.

Kosmin, Barry A., Ariela Keysar, Ryan Cragun, and Juhem Navarro-Rivera. *American Nones: The Profile of the "No Religion" Population*. Hartford, CT: The American Religious Identify Survey Project, Trinity College, 2008.

Larson, Edward J. and Larry Witham. "Scientists Are Still Keeping the Faith." *Nature* 386, no. 6624 (1997): 435–436.

Leuba, James. *The Belief in God and Immortality: A Psychological, Anthropological, and Statistical Study*. Chicago: Open Court Publishers, 1921.

Marcus, Jacob R. *Early American Jewry: The Jews of New York, New England, and Canada, 1649–1794: Volume I*. Philadelphia: Jewish Publication Society, 1951.

Masco, Joseph. "Atomic Health, or How the Bomb Altered American Notions of Death." In *Against Health: How Health Became the New Morality*, eds. Jonathan M. Metzl, and Anna Kirkland, 133–154. New York: NYU Press, 2010.

McDougall, Walter A. *Promised Land, Crusader State: The American Encounter with the World Since 1776*. New York: Houghton Mifflin, 1997.

Mehta, Nalin and Upahar Pramanik. "HIV and the Gurus: Religiosity, Plurality and the Challenge of a 'Hindu" Response." *South Asian History and Culture* 1, no. 2 (2010): 250–267.

Mohler, Albert. "Where Have All the Liberals Gone?—The Riverside Church Seeks New Pastor." albertmohler.com, May 9, 2007. www.albertmohler.com/2007/05/09/where-have-all-the-liberals-gone-the-riverside-church-seeks-new-pastor/. Accessed February 28, 2018.

Mohler, Albert. "The Southern Baptist Convention and the Issue of Interdenominational Partnerships." Memorandum, Louisville, KY, 2009. https://albertmohler.com/2009/07/16/the-southern-baptist-convention-and-the-issue-of-interdenominational-relationships/. Accessed March 7, 2018.

Nurser, John. "The 'Ecumenical Movement' Churches, 'Global Order,' and Human Rights: 1938–1948." *Human Rights Quarterly* 25, no. 4 (2003): 841–881.

Olivier, Jill. "'An FB-oh?': Mapping the Etymology of the Religious Entity Engaged in Health." In *When Religion and Health Align: Mobilizing Religious Health Assets for Transformation*, eds. James Cochrane, Barbara Schmid, and Teresa Cutts. Pietermaritzburg, SA: Cluster Publications, 2011.

Pew Research Center. Faith on the Hill: Religious Composition of the 114th Congress. Washington, DC: Pew Research Center, 2015. www.pewforum.org/2015/01/05/faith-on-the-hill/. Accessed March 4, 2018.

Pew Research Center. "America's Changing Religious Landscape." Washington, DC: Pew Research Center, 2015. http://assets.pewresearch.org/wp-content/uploads/sites/11/2015/05/RLS-08-26-full-report.pdf. Accessed March 5, 2018.

"Protest to Eisenhower: Group Asks Him to Reconsider Speech to Church Council." *The New York Times*, August 7, 1954, p. 14.

Schlumpf, Heidi. "Gregory Baum, Influential Theologian of Vatican II Era, Dies at 94." *National Catholic Reporter*, October 20, 2017. www.ncronline.org/news/people/gregory-baum-influential-theologian-vatican-ii-era-dies-94. Accessed March 5, 2018.

Southern Baptist Convention. "Resolution on Abortion." Resolution, St. Louis, MO, 1971. www.sbc.net/resolutions/13/resolution-on-abortion. Accessed March 7, 2018.

Stark, Rodney. "Secularization, R.I.P." *Sociology of Religion* 60, no. 3 (1999): 249–273.

U.S. Conference of Catholic Bishops. *Sharing Catholic Social Teaching: Challenges and Directions—Reflections of the U.S. Bishops*. Washington, DC: USCCB Publishing, 1998.

United States Census Bureau. "Section I: Population." Statistical Abstract of the United States: 2012 (131st Edition), Washington: U.S. Census Bureau, 2012. www.census.gov/library/publications/2011/compendia/statab/131ed/population.html. Accessed March 5, 2018.

8 Not "either/or" but "both/and"

On seeing international health and development as a tragic profession . . . and why that should give us hope

The reader who has plowed through the last seven chapters has been privy to a dizzying array of vignettes illustrating the relationship between American Protestant Christian and global health and development. Those relationships are complex and contradictory. I would ask that those who have only undertaken a more cursory read grant me a moment to recount just a few of those vignettes to give some context to this last chapter.

Anne Hutchinson, that skilled midwife of the Massachusetts Bay Colony, was banished from her community in 1638 for daring to question the authority of the male religious leaders of her church by describing the nature of God's grace for their tastes. As it developed in the United States, that same religious tradition provided a place for women to assume key leadership in the only context in which global health could be practiced for decades—foreign missions. Dr. Clara Swain was the first woman sent by Protestant Americans on medical mission; she was sent to India in 1869 where she established a nurse's colleges that graduated its first class in 1873. Dr. Lucinda Combs followed not long after in 1872, traveling to China, where the medical facilities she established were credited with saving the life of a senior Chinese leader. With these first leaders, the "doors were thrown open [to women in medical missions] and thousands of others followed."[1] By 1910, 55% of all the American staff involved in Protestant medical missions were women.[2] Women working today in global health and development, regardless of their religious faith or absence of faith, are connected to the "both/and" of this history of Protestantism if, indeed, the main thesis is correct in claiming that present-day global health and development institutions and practices have been influenced by a secularized "in-depth Christianity" carried forth by these very missionaries.

In 1721, Puritan minister Cotton Mather, called for all British inhabitants of Massachusetts to be inoculated against smallpox. "Anti-vaxxers" were in force even then; one of them throw a small explosive device into Mather's home (it didn't explode) yelling, "Cotton Mather, you dog, dam you! I'll inoculate you with this; with a pox to you!" Public health advocates who would cheer Mather's foresight must also remember his words about the Native Americans whose land he and the follow colonist had stolen—Mather believed "that it would be the most unexceptionable piece of justice in the world for to extinguish the offending savages."

The earliest and most ardent religious champions of contraception were the religious leaders of liberal Protestant denominations. These leaders were clear supporters of the Social Gospel—and of eugenics. Their moral commitment to addressing social, economic, and health inequity also led them to support making contraceptive technologies available to racial minorities, the poor, and "the feeble-minded" while also exhorting the husbands and wives in their all-white congregations to have more children all in an effort to prevent the "race suicide" of the Anglo-Saxon people. These same racist opinions are found both in the Social Gospel writings of Josiah Strong and in the words of John Shaw Billings, early public health pioneer and one of the founders of the American Public Health Association.

British Protestants who came to America spoke eloquently about religious freedom but when the nation's first national congressional body, the Continental Congress, convened for the first time in 1774, the body's first act was to condemn the British Parliament for granting Catholics in the Quebec Province of Canada the freedom to assemble and worship. George Angier Gordon, pastor at Old South Church in Boston, preaching a sermon entitled "The Gospel for Humanity" at the 1895 meeting of the American Board of Commissioners for Foreign Mission said that,

> Jesus must prove himself a better ruler to Japan, a nobler Confucius to China, a diviner Gautama to India; the whole sacred past must reappear in Him utterly transfigured and carried utterly beyond itself. . . . He must come as the consummation of the ideals of every nation under Heaven.[3]

Religious freedom and tolerance, it seems, were largely reserved for Christians, and only certain kinds of Christian at that.

In 2010, William Jenkins, a public health legend in America who has provided leadership on health initiatives for African American communities for decades, described to the participants at the Annual Meeting of the American Public Health Association the elements of a longitudinal epidemiological study that demonstrated ideal characteristics of community-based participatory research. Public health practitioners who are committed to feasible, sustainable public health models that value and respect communities' insights, resources, capacities, and contributions will be dismayed to know that Dr. Jenkins was describing the Tuskegee Syphilis Study.[4] Jenkins's point, obviously, was not to praise the study but to remind us that our current approaches to public health practice are not immune to the kinds of violent dehumanization characterized by the four decade study.

The message of America's civil religion justified the Spanish-American War as Social Gospel leaders proclaimed "that if it be the will of Almighty God that by war the last trace of this inhumanity of man to man shall be swept away from this

Western hemisphere, let it come!" The same religious rhetoric of America's destiny to be an instrument in God's plan for the salvation of the world was repeated in the "progressive imperialism" that justified the occupation of the Philippines and other former Spanish territories, even after the citizens there rose up in rebellion against our presence and fought against American forces—a conflict that cost 200,000 Filipino their lives. That same rhetoric provided a rationale for the nation to commit to a comprehensive, sustained public health and education initiative in the nation.

Researchers with the U.S. Public Health Service carried out the Tuskegee experiments and a similar set of experiments in Guatemala to better understand the etiology, prevention, and treatment of syphilis. In Guatemala, public health researchers intentionally exposed people who weren't infected to syphilis in an effort to search for an effective prevention approach for American soldiers.

These examples briefly recounted here serve as reminders that religion, health, and development are all serious endeavors. As sources of knowledge and foundations for practice, each of these things call those of us who place our trust in them to make wagers fraught with moral weight about the best ways to organize our institutions and societies to eradicate disease, make opportunities more widely available, level the playing field, and move us toward a more just and humane world. The reason such wagers are fraught is not because of the intentions behind them but because of the very real possibility of our delusion. Such possibilities of delusion are real because the examples of such delusions are abundant in each of these fields, as the vignettes above illustrate. So what, pray tell, do we do about our delusions?

In Chapters 4 and 5, I developed the concepts of the social evangelist, the social engineer, and the social reconstructionist to describe the ways in which a secularized Social Gospel had helped to establish key elements of global health and development work. Those two chapters provided seven short case studies of the evangelist, engineer, reconstructionist, evangelist/engineer, evangelist/reconstructionist, engineer/reconstructionist, and evangelist/engineer/reconstructionist. In reality, of course, such separations may not be very helpful. The fact is that the people profiled in each of those examples moved across each of the positions of the reconstructionist, the evangelist, and the engineer.

The fields of global health and development and the newly-emerging sub-discipline of religion and public health desperately need to adopt a tri-focal lens of evangelist, engineer, and reconstructionist. On an ongoing basis. And, simultaneously. Such adoption needs to be across the fields and not merely as a focus of random clusters of individual researchers or practitioners; in other words, we all need to gain some capacity to function in these roles. We need to adopt these lenses precisely because the social networks upon which global health and development are built are marked by intricate, intersecting interests and priorities. Religion resides within those networks, as do other social and political forces. We need to spot when power is operative within these networks that will thwart health rather than further it. Perhaps more importantly, we need to spot when power is operative within these networks to improve circumstances for some (including health and economic opportunity) by compromising it for others. And when we sport such power, we need to resist and refuse it.

This may sound rather self-evident and straightforward. It isn't. In fact, it is inordinately difficult, especially for fields such as global health and development which are so reliant on revenue streams from governments and civil society to carry out essential work and keep hard-working, dedicated, idealistic people employed. Such funding always comes with strings—political interests or research focuses and methodologies that may be at odds with the people who will be the subjects of a given project. Saying no to such power is difficult, even when we prospectively see it. Finding ways to extricate ourselves from that kind of power when we're already directly implicated in it is exponentially harder. This is why we need the prophetic call of the reconstructionist to call out misplaced priorities and self-deluded justifications. It is why we need the engineer to help us develop feasible, sustainable, relevant programs that will actually reflect the needs and priorities of local communities. It is why we need the evangelist to remind us what our commitments are as we go up against so many distracting forces.

Standing in the intersection of these three frameworks is a tall order. It will likely drive the evidence-driven engineer crazy. How can you ever do that? Is it feasible? Where's your proof of the need? What method would you employ? How would you evaluate the process, the outcomes, the impact? Such questions are legitimate but beyond the scope of this book. Nonetheless, I would argue that such an approach is needed because *what we're doing isn't working*. At least, it's "not working" far too often.

The engineer is not the only one with reservations. The reconstructionist is wary of taking things to scale, suspicious of becoming part of the systems and structures and mechanisms, afraid of being co-opted. Again, this reservation is understandable. And while I would argue that the iconoclastic reconstructionist can avoid certain ethical compromises by staying out of such entanglements, in my experience more of us want to employ the rhetoric of the reconstructionist even while strolling through the halls of power. The would-be reconstructionists among us must be honest about the subject position we occupy and ask ourselves whether we are really, truly that iconoclastic. Many of us drawn to the reconstructionist frameworks delude ourselves regarding the extent and purity of our radicalism even as we stay ensconced in institutions of social power and privilege with their attendant salaries.

Finally, the evangelist may resist this call because she simply wants to share the good news of health. The problem with such an approach alone is that it is naïve. Public health and development happen at social scale beyond the individual and for those of us from cultures such as the U.S., they involve an intervention into another culture (think about that word for a moment—intervention) at a societal level. From our point of view, we may be bringing good news (the very definition of evangelism) even as those who are the "target populations" of our intervention see our work as the newest chapter in the saga of empire. Global health and development initiatives—whether faith-based or secular—can have elements of either; most of the time they have elements of both.

When liberal Protestants adopted the roles of social reconstructionist, social evangelist, and social engineer to implement elements of the Social Gospel in secular institutions during the middle decades of the twentieth century, their social power decreased. The same may occur for global health and development practitioners—not because we have nothing to say but because we may say things that most people don't want to hear.

To gain some perspective to see through all three lenses simultaneously, global health researchers and practitioners need to acknowledge our own cultural particularity. We travel halfway around the world and carry out formative research to gather insights into the cultures of the places where we work but we rarely articulate the cultural assumptions underwriting our own efforts. Most of us are victims of the social iatrogenesis described by Illich (see Chapter 4) in which we've lost other narratives to make sense of our work outside of the frameworks of modern public health and development practice. Further, any effort to remember those other narratives will require us to interrogate our own cultural iatrogenesis also described by Illich—we'll have to recognize that many people in many societies in many parts of the world already live in and operate out of different narratives of health from the ones that purport to tell those of us in global health research and practice the truth.

Finally, we would do well to remember that our health and development practices sometimes place us in tragic positions. In saying that, I am not only referring to the fact that global health and development work means experiencing illness, poverty, and disparities playing out not only in individuals' lives but across societies, sometimes in places with glaring health, social, and economic challenges. Rather, I am referring to the tragedy that is hard-wired into the fundamental goal of health for all people in all societies. We have set for ourselves this impossible goal and we find ourselves working mightily to achieve it. The impossibility of our goals could only be achieved by working across myriad social and political institutions that are by their very definition at odds with one another. In short, they really are impossible; that doesn't mean we don't stop striving.

The systems within which we operate will at times place us in a position where the health and social benefits we so desperately desire can only be achieved in a significant portion of a population by another part of the population paying a price. Finding ourselves in such instances in which somebody pays that price because of our work is what I mean by the tragic nature of global health and development practice. In such circumstances, some system of intense moral reflection would be immensely helpful. Of all the contributions that the new-found interest in religion could provide to the field of global health and development, this may be the most profound and the most needed.

This is not to say that religious traditions are the only systems through which one may be schooled in the methods for moral reflection—there are certainly others. It is not to say that such a religious system is qualitatively better in providing moral honesty and clarity than a secular one—there is no way to measure that *a priori*. But it is to say that any tradition by its very nature is a source of knowledge that contains a history and takes that history seriously. As such, it will contain narratives over the course of its history that speak to this conundrum, this paradox. And yes, this tragedy. Global health and development would do well to read such narratives—many of which will be religious—and learn from them because we only want to tell the history of our work in the glossy pages of annual reports that show smiling mothers and well-fed children.

Even when we demonstrate a frightening capacity to carry out an intervention or study that in retrospect is unconscionable in its assumptions as in the case of the Tuskegee study, we assume that new methodologies of ethical review and clearance—new mechanisms and steps in our SOPs—will prevent us from repeating such violence. We are ill-equipped to acknowledge the tragic dimensions of our work because we are part of a culture within health and development practice that can't tell those aspects of our own story. Religious traditions that tell the truth of their own tragic collusion with power and violence—collusion that was rationalized and justified in the name of God—could give us some courage to face our own truths.

Sometimes, our health and development practice will produce both good and bad consequences at the same time. Under such circumstances, we simply don't have the ways to reflect on whether the choice to undertake the action is right or wrong; the tradition of bioethics that ground most public health ethics is employed in mechanistic frameworks that simply can't account for this scenario. This is what we can't disentangle: good and right, bad and wrong. We can't disentangle these things because we can't acknowledge that our practices might result in bad consequences. The failure to acknowledge this leaves us in a dangerous situation.

One step in addressing such a failure would include creating communities within global health and development that tell a fuller, better, more accurate and true story of what's at stake than what is currently possible through our logic models enumerating impacts, protocols spelling out our efforts to shield vulnerable subjects from risk, outcome evaluations that show us what we accomplished, and retrospective assessments of unexpected outcomes that would have been foreseeable.

In short, perhaps the first step in our work would be to quit pretending that success in Health for All 2000, or Healthy People 2020, or the Millennium Development Goals, or the Sustainable Development Goals, or HIV Fast Track, or Partnership for an HIV-Free Generation is the necessary precursor to the promised land of a medical and social utopia. What would happen if we acknowledged that we have never met such goals and objectives and that we can't meet them for all people in all places at all times—which doesn't mean that our efforts expended toward those goals have failed to contribute to improved health and social outcomes. What would happen if we gave up on the criterion of (impossible) success and opted instead for sticking with communities not through the duration of our funding stream but as the hallmark of true relationships? What if we gave up on the idea of transferring the empire of the world to America or to other countries through the exceptional role that America continues telling itself it is destined to play? What if we gave up on the idea of empire and its transfer altogether?

The possibility of giving up on empire in the social and political systems that comprise our world today is as illusory as achieving 100% compliance to the Sustainable Development Goals. This is why we need a way to narrate the tragic aspects of our work to keep us honest and avoid the tendency to see ourselves as modern saints. The failure of the Social Gospel to Christianize the social order required liberal Protestants to develop a strong and vibrant strand of reconstruction in the aftermath of its tragic collapse. That collapse was not the same as its failure. In the aftermath, various theological traditions of social analysis and critique emerged, as we discussed in Chapter 5. This reconstructionist strand is desperately needed within the field of global health and development. By providing a social history of religion and health and demonstrating that such history is riddled with instances of complexities and contradictions, of tragedy and tenacity, perhaps this book will make a small contribution in that regard.

Notes

1 I am not citing the sources for these vignettes, since those sources were cited in the earlier chapters. The only citations will be for elements in the vignettes not originally recounted in the earlier sections of the book. Walter Lambuth, *Medical Missions: The Two-Fold Task* (New York: Student Volunteer Movement for Medical Missions, 1920), 136–137.

2 William R. Hutchison, *Errand to the World: American Protestant Thought and Foreign Missions* (Chicago: University of Chicago Press, 1987), 101.

3 Ibid., p. 106.

4 William Jenkins, *Opening Plenary of the American Public Health Association* (speech, Denver, CO, November 7, 2010), www.youtube.com/watch?v=BragfuSDoow, accessed March 15, 2017.

References

Douthat, Ross. "Can Liberal Christianity Be Saved?" *The New York Times*, July 15, 2012, p. SR11.

Hutchison, William R. *Errand to the World: American Protestant Thought and Foreign Missions*. Chicago: University of Chicago Press, 1987.

Jenkins, William. "Opening Plenary of the American Public Health Association." Speech, Denver, CO, November 7, 2010. www.youtube.com/watch?v=BragfuSDoow. Accessed March 15, 2017.

Lambuth, Walter. *Medical Missions: The Two-Fold Task*. New York: Student Volunteer Movement for Medical Missions, 1920.

Index

CPSIA information can be obtained
at www.ICGtesting.com
Printed in the USA
LVHW081531030922
727559LV00003B/114

9 780815 356738